Virtual Clinical Excursions—General Hospital

for

Harkreader, Hogan, and Thobaben
Fundamentals of Nursing:
Caring and Clinical Judgment,
3rd Edition

Virtual Clinical Excursions—General Hospital

for

Harkreader, Hogan, and Thobaben
Fundamentals of Nursing:
Caring and Clinical Judgment,
3rd Edition

prepared by

Kim D. Cooper, RN, MSN
Ivy Tech Community College
Terre Haute, Indiana

software developed by
Wolfsong Informatics, LLC
Tucson, Arizona

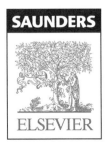

SAUNDERS

ELSEVIER

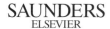

SAUNDERS
ELSEVIER

11830 Westline Industrial Dr.
St. Louis, Missouri 63146

VIRTUAL CLINICAL EXCURSIONS—GENERAL HOSPITAL FOR
HARKREADER, HOGAN, AND THOBABEN
FUNDAMENTALS OF NURSING: CARING AND CLINICAL JUDGMENT
THIRD EDITION

ISBN: 978-1-4160-4459-8

Notice

Knowledge and best practice in this field are constantly changing. As new research and experience broaden our knowledge, changes in practice, treatment and drug therapy may become necessary or appropriate. Readers are advised to check the most current information provided (i) on procedures featured or (ii) by the manufacturer of each product to be administered, to verify the recommended dose or formula, the method and duration of administration, and contraindications. It is the responsibility of the practitioner, relying on their own experience and knowledge of the patient, to make diagnoses, to determine dosages and the best treatment for each individual patient, and to take all appropriate safety precautions. To the fullest extent of the law, neither the Publisher nor the Authors assumes any liability for any injury and/or damage to persons or property arising out or related to any use of the material contained in this book.

ISBN: 978-1-4160-4459-8

Executive Editor: *Tom Wilhelm*
Managing Editor: *Jeff Downing*
Associate Developmental Editor: *Tiffany Trautwein*
Book Production Manager: *Gayle May*
Project Manager: *Tracey Schriefer*

Printed in the United States of America

Last digit is the print number: 9 8 7 6 5 4 3 2 1

Workbook
prepared by

Kim D. Cooper, RN, MSN
Ivy Tech Community College
Terre Haute, Indiana

Textbook

Helen Harkreader, PhD, RN
Professor
Austin Community College
Austin, Texas

Mary Ann Hogan, RN, MSN
Clinical Assistant Professor
School of Nursing
University of Massachusetts Amherst
Amherst, Massachusetts

Marshelle Thobaben, MS, RN, PHN, APNP, FNP
Professor and
Community Health and Psychiatric Nursing Consultant
Department of Nursing
Humboldt State University
Arcata, California

Reviewer

Gina Long, RN, DNSc
Assistant Professor, Department of Nursing
College of Health Professions
Northern Arizona University
Flagstaff, Arizona

Contents

Table of Contents
Harkreader, Hogan, Thobaben:
Fundamentals of Nursing, 3rd Edition

Getting Started

GETTING SET UP

■ MINIMUM SYSTEM REQUIREMENTS

WINDOWS™

Windows XP, 2000, 98, ME, NT 4.0 (Recommend Windows XP/2000)
Pentium® III processor (or equivalent) @ 600 MHz (Recommend 800 MHz or better)
128 MB of RAM (Recommend 256 MB or more)
800 x 600 screen size (Recommend 1024 x 768)
Thousands of colors
12x CD-ROM drive
Soundblaster 16 soundcard compatibility
Stereo speakers or headphones

Note: Virtual Clinical Excursions—General Hospital for Windows will require a minimal amount of disk space to install icons and required dll files for Windows 98/ME.

MACINTOSH®

MAC OS X (10.2 or higher)
Apple Power PC G3 @ 500 MHz or better
128 MB of RAM (Recommend 256 MB or more)
800 x 600 screen size (Recommend 1024 x 768)
Thousands of colors
12x CD-ROM drive
Stereo speakers or headphones

■ INSTALLATION INSTRUCTIONS

WINDOWS

1. Insert the *Virtual Clinical Excursions—General Hospital* CD-ROM.
2. Inserting the CD should automatically bring up the setup screen if the current product is not already installed.
   a. If the setup screen does not appear automatically (and *Virtual Clinical Excursions— General Hospital* has not been installed already), navigate to the "My Computer" icon on your desktop or in your Start menu.
   b. Double-click on your CD-ROM drive.
   c. If installation does not start at this point:
      (1) Click the **Start** icon on the task bar and select the **Run** option.
      (2) Type d:\setup.exe (where "d:\" is your CD-ROM drive) and press **OK**.
      (3) Follow the onscreen instructions for installation.
3. Follow the onscreen instructions during the setup process.

MACINTOSH

1. Insert the *Virtual Clinical Excursions—General Hospital* CD in the CD-ROM drive. The disk icon will appear on your desktop.
2. Double-click on the disk icon.
3. Double-click on the GENERAL-HOSPITAL_MAC run file.

Note: Virtual Clinical Excursions—General Hospital for Macintosh does not have an installation setup and can only be run directly from the CD.

■ HOW TO USE VIRTUAL CLINICAL EXCURSIONS—GENERAL HOSPITAL

WINDOWS

1. Double-click on the *Virtual Clinical Excursions—General Hospital* icon located on your desktop.
2. Or navigate to the program via the Windows Start menu.

Note: Windows 98/ME will require you to restart your computer before running the *Virtual Clinical Excursions—General Hospital* program.

MACINTOSH

1. Insert the *Virtual Clinical Excursions—General Hospital* CD in the CD-ROM drive. The disk icon will appear on your desktop.
2. Double-click on the disk icon.
3. Double-click on the GENERAL-HOSPITAL_MAC run file.

■ SCREEN SETTINGS

For best results, your computer monitor resolution should be set at a minimum of 800 x 600. The number of colors displayed should be set to "thousands or higher" (High Color or 16 bit) or "millions of colors" (True Color or 24 bit).

Windows™

1. From the **Start** menu, select **Control Panel** (on some systems, you will first go to **Settings**, then to **Control Panel**).
2. Double-click on the **Display** icon.
3. Click on the **Settings** tab.
4. Under **Screen resolution** use the slider bar to select **800 by 600 pixels**.
5. Access the **Colors** drop-down menu by clicking on the down arrow.
6. Select **High Color (16 bit)** or **True Color (24 bit)**.
7. Click on **OK**.
8. You may be asked to verify the setting changes. Click **Yes**.
9. You may be asked to restart your computer to accept the changes. Click **Yes**.

Macintosh®

1. Select the **Monitors** control panel.
2. Select **800 x 600** (or similar) from the **Resolution** area.
3. Select **Thousands** or **Millions** from the **Color Depth** area.

■ WEB BROWSERS

Supported web browsers include Microsoft Internet Explorer (IE) version 6.0 or higher, Netscape version 7.1 or higher, and Mozilla Firefox version 1.4 or higher.

If you use America Online (AOL) for web access, you will need AOL version 4.0 or higher and IE 5.0 or higher. Do not use earlier versions of AOL with earlier versions of IE, because you will have difficulty accessing many features.

For best results with AOL:
- Connect to the Internet using AOL version 4.0 or higher.
- Open a private chat within AOL (this allows the AOL client to remain open, without asking whether you wish to disconnect while minimized).
- Minimize AOL.
- Launch a recommended browser.

■ TECHNICAL SUPPORT

Technical support for this product is available between 7:30 a.m. and 7 p.m. (CST), Monday through Friday. Before calling, be sure that your computer meets the minimum system requirements to run this software. Inside the United States and Canada, call 1-800-692-9010. Outside North America, call 314-872-8370. You may also fax your questions to 314-523-4932 or contact Technical Support through e-mail: technical.support@elsevier.com.

Trademarks: Windows, Macintosh, Pentium, and America Online are registered trademarks.

ACCESSING *Virtual Clinical Excursions—General-Hospital* FROM EVOLVE

The product you have purchased is part of the Evolve family of online courses and learning resources. Please read the following information thoroughly to get started.

To access your instructor's course on Evolve:

Your instructor will provide you with the username and password needed to access this specific course on the Evolve Learning System. Once you have received this information, please follow these instructions:

1. Go to the Evolve student page (http://evolve.elsevier.com/student)

2. Enter your username and password in the **Login to My Evolve** area and click the **Login** button.

3. You will be taken to your personalized **My Evolve** page, where the course will be listed in the **My Courses** module.

TECHNICAL REQUIREMENTS

To use an Evolve course, you will need access to a computer that is connected to the Internet and equipped with web browser software that supports frames. For optimal performance, it is recommended that you have speakers and use a high-speed Internet connection. However, slower dial-up modems (56 K minimum) are acceptable.

Whichever browser you use, the browser preferences must be set to enable cookies and JavaScript and the cache must be set to reload every time.

Enable Cookies

Browser	Steps
Internet Explorer (IE) 6.0 or higher	1. Select **Tools → Internet Options**. 2. Select **Privacy** tab. 3. Use the slider (slide down) to **Accept All Cookies**. 4. Click **OK**. -OR- 3. Click the **Advanced** button. 4. Click the check box next to **Override Automatic Cookie Handling**. 5. Click the **Accept** radio buttons under **First-party Cookies** and **Third-party Cookies**. 6. Click **OK**.
Netscape 7.1 or higher	1. Select **Edit → Preferences**. 2. Select **Privacy & Security**. 3. Select **Cookies**. 4. Select **Enable All Cookies**.
Mozilla Firefox 1.4 or higher	1. Select **Tools → Options**. 2. Select the **Privacy** icon. 3. Click to expand Cookies. 4. Select **Allow sites to set cookies**. 5. Click **OK**.

Enable JavaScript

Browser	Steps
Internet Explorer (IE) 6.0 or higher	1. Select **Tools → Internet Options**. 2. Select **Security** tab. 3. Under **Security level for this zone** set to **Medium** or lower.
Netscape 7.1 or higher	1. Select **Edit → Preferences**. 2. Select **Advanced**. 3. Select **Scripts & Plugins**. 4. Make sure the **Navigator** box is checked to **Enable JavaScript**. 5. Click **OK**.
Mozilla Firefox 1.4 or higher	1. Select **Tools → Options**. 2. Select the **Content** icon. 3. Select **Enable JavaScript**. 4. Click **OK**.

Set Cache to Always Reload a Page

Browser	Steps
Internet Explorer (IE) 6.0 or higher	1. Select **Tools → Internet Options**. 2. Select **General** tab. 3. Go to the **Temporary Internet Files** and click the **Settings** button. 4. Select the radio button for **Every visit to the page** and click **OK** when complete.
Netscape 7.1 or higher	1. Select **Edit → Preferences**. 2. Select **Advanced**. 3. Select **Cache**. 4. Select the **Every time I view the page** radio button. 5. Click **OK**.
Mozilla Firefox 1.4 or higher	1. Select **Tools → Options**. 2. Select the **Privacy** icon. 3. Click to expand Cache. 4. Set the value to "**0**" in the **Use up to: __ MB of disk space for the cache** field. 5. Click **OK**.

Plug-Ins

Adobe Acrobat Reader—With the free Acrobat Reader software, you can view and print Adobe PDF files. Many Evolve products offer student and instructor manuals, checklists, and more in this format!

Download at: http://www.adobe.com

Apple QuickTime—Install this to hear word pronunciations, heart and lung sounds, and many other helpful audio clips within Evolve Online Courses!

Download at: http://www.apple.com

Adobe Flash Player—This player will enhance your viewing of many Evolve web pages, as well as educational short-form to long-form animation within the Evolve Learning System!

Download at: http://www.adobe.com

Adobe Shockwave Player—Shockwave is best for viewing the many interactive learning activities within Evolve Online Courses!

Download at: http://www.adobe.com

Microsoft Word Viewer—With this viewer Microsoft Word users can share documents with those who don't have Word, and users without Word can open and view Word documents. Many Evolve products have testbank, student and instructor manuals, and other documents available for downloading and viewing on your own computer!

Download at: http://www.microsoft.com

Microsoft PowerPoint Viewer—View PowerPoint 97, 2000, and 2002 presentations even if you don't have PowerPoint with this viewer. Many Evolve products have slides available for downloading and viewing on your own computer!

Download at: http://www.microsoft.com

SUPPORT INFORMATION

Live support is available to customers in the United States and Canada from 7:30 a.m. to 7 p.m. (CST), Monday through Friday by calling **1-800-401-9962**. You can also send an email to evolve-support@elsevier.com.

There is also **24/7 support information** available on the Evolve website (http://evolve.elsevier.com), including:

- Guided Tours
- Tutorials
- Frequently Asked Questions (FAQs)
- Online Copies of Course User Guides
- And much more!

A QUICK TOUR

Welcome to *Virtual Clinical Excursions—General Hospital*, a virtual hospital setting in which you can work with multiple complex patient simulations and also learn to access and evaluate the information resources that are essential for high-quality patient care. The virtual hospital, Pacific View Regional Hospital, has realistic architecture and access to patient rooms, a Nurses' Station, and a Medication Room.

■ BEFORE YOU START

Make sure you have your textbook nearby when you use the *Virtual Clinical Excursions—General Hospital* CD. You will want to consult topic areas in your textbook frequently while working with the CD and using this workbook.

■ HOW TO SIGN IN

- Enter your name on the Student Nurse identification badge.
- Next, specify the floor on which you will work. The Medical-Surgical Floor is automatically chosen next to **Select Floor**. If you wish to select another floor (Skilled Nursing or Obstetrics), click the down arrow to access the menu. For this quick tour, choose the Medical-Surgical Floor.
- Now click the down arrow next to **Select Period of Care**. This drop-down menu gives you four periods of care from which to choose. In Periods of Care 1 through 3, you can actively engage in patient assessment, entry of data in the electronic patient record (EPR), and medication administration. Period of Care 4 presents the day in review. Highlight and click the appropriate period of care. (For this quick tour, choose **Period of Care 1**.) Click **Go**. This takes you to the Patient List screen (see example on page 11). Only the patients on the floor you choose (Medical-Surgical) are available. Note that the virtual time is provided in the box at the lower left corner of the screen (0730, since we chose Period of Care 1).

Note: If you choose to work during Period of Care 4: 1900-2000, the Patient List screen is skipped since you are not able to visit patients or administer medications during the shift. Instead, you are taken directly to the Nurses' Station, where the records of all the patients on the floor are available for your review.

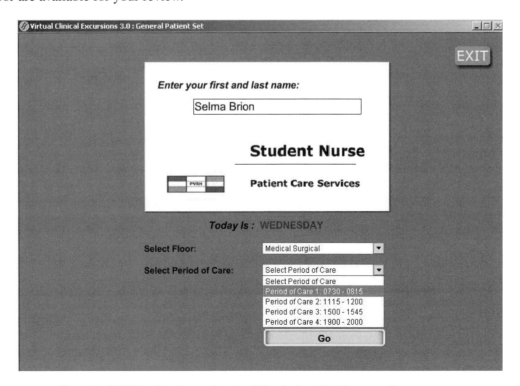

■ **PATIENT LIST**

MEDICAL-SURGICAL UNIT

Harry George (Room 401)
Osteomyelitis—A 54-year-old Caucasian male admitted from a homeless shelter with an infected leg. He has complications of type 2 diabetes mellitus, alcohol abuse, nicotine addiction, poor pain control, and complex psychosocial issues.

Jacquline Catanazaro (Room 402)
Asthma—A 45-year-old Caucasian female admitted with an acute asthma exacerbation and suspected pneumonia. She has complications of chronic schizophrenia, noncompliance with medication therapy, obesity, and herniated disc.

Piya Jordan (Room 403)
Bowel obstruction—A 68-year-old Asian female admitted with a colon mass and suspected adenocarcinoma. She undergoes a right hemicolectomy. This patient's complications include atrial fibrillation, hypokalemia, and symptoms of meperidine toxicity.

Clarence Hughes (Room 404)
Degenerative joint disease—A 73-year-old African-American male admitted for a left total knee replacement. His preparations for discharge are complicated by the development of a pulmonary embolus and the need for ongoing intravenous therapy.

Pablo Rodriguez (Room 405)
Metastatic lung carcinoma—A 71-year-old Hispanic male admitted with symptoms of dehydration and malnutrition. He has chronic pain secondary to multiple subcutaneous skin nodules and psychosocial concerns related to family issues with his approaching death.

Patricia Newman (Room 406)
Pneumonia—A 61-year-old Caucasian female admitted with worsening pulmonary function and an acute respiratory infection. Her chronic emphysema is complicated by heavy smoking, hypertension, and malnutrition. She needs access to community resources such as a smoking cessation program and meal assistance.

SKILLED NURSING UNIT

William Jefferson (Room 501)
Alzheimer's disease—A 75-year-old African-American male admitted for stabilization of type 2 diabetes and hypertension following a recent acute care admission for a urinary tract infection and sepsis. His complications include episodes of acute delirium and a history of osteoarthritis.

Kathryn Doyle (Room 503)
Rehabilitation post left hip replacement—A 79-year-old Caucasian female admitted following a complicated recovery from an ORIF. She is experiencing symptoms of malnutrition and depression due to unstable family dynamics, placing her at risk for elder abuse.

Goro Oishi (Room 505)
Hospice care—A 66-year-old Asian male admitted following an acute care admission for an intracerebral hemorrhage and resulting coma. Family-staff interactions provide opportunities to explore death and dying issues related to conflict about advanced life support and cultural and religious differences.

OBSTETRICS UNIT

Dorothy Grant (Room 201)
30-week intrauterine pregnancy—A 25-year-old multipara admitted with abdominal trauma following a domestic violence incident. Her complications include preterm labor and extensive social issues such as acquiring safe housing for her family upon discharge.

■ HOW TO SELECT A PATIENT

- You can choose one or more patients to work with from the Patient List by checking the box to the left of the patient name(s). For this quick tour, select Piya Jordan and Pablo Rodriguez. (In order to receive a scorecard for a patient, the patient must be selected before proceeding to the Nurses' Station.)
- Click on **Get Report** to the right of the medical records number (MRN) to view a summary of the patient's care during the 12-hour period before your arrival on the unit.
- After reviewing the report, click on **Go to Nurses' Station** in the right lower corner to begin your care. (*Note:* If you have been assigned to care for multiple patients, you can click on **Return to Patient List** to select and review the report for each additional patient before going to the Nurses' Station.)

Note: Even though the Patient List is initially skipped when you sign in to work for Period of Care 4, you can still access this screen if you wish to review the shift-change report for any of the patients. To do so, simply click on **Patient List** near the top left corner of the Nurses' Station (or click on the clipboard to the left of the Kardex). Then click on **Get Report** for the patient(s) whose care you are reviewing. This may be done during any period of care.

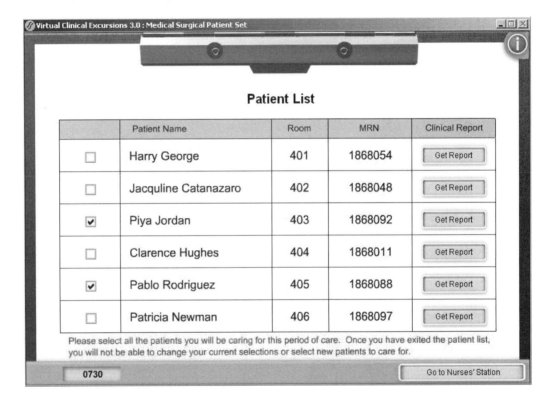

■ HOW TO FIND A PATIENT'S RECORDS

NURSES' STATION

Within the Nurses' Station, you will see:

1. A clipboard that contains the patient list for that floor.
2. A chart rack with patient charts labeled by room number, a notebook labeled Kardex, and a notebook labeled MAR (Medication Administration Record).
3. A desktop computer with access to the Electronic Patient Record (EPR).
4. A tool bar across the top of the screen that can also be used to access the Patient List, EPR, Chart, MAR, and Kardex. This tool bar is also accessible from each patient's room.
5. A Drug Guide containing information about the medications you are able to administer to your patients.
6. A tool bar across the bottom of the screen that you can use to access patient rooms, the Medication Room, the Floor Map, or the Drug Guide.

As you run your cursor over an item, it will be highlighted. To select, simply double-click on the item. As you use these resources, you will always be able to return to the Nurses' Station by clicking on the **Return to Nurses' Station** bar located in the right lower corner of your screen.

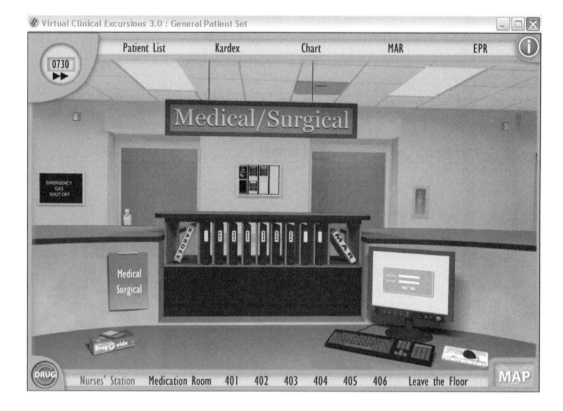

MEDICATION ADMINISTRATION RECORD (MAR)

The MAR icon located in the tool bar at the top of your screen accesses current 24-hour medications for each patient. Click on the icon and the MAR will open. (*Note:* You can also access the MAR by clicking on the MAR notebook on the far right side of the book rack in the center of the screen.) Within the MAR, tabs on the right side of the screen allow you to select patients by room number. Be careful to make sure you select the correct tab number for *your* patient rather than simply reading the first record that appears after the MAR opens. Each MAR sheet lists the following:

- Medications
- Route and dosage of each medication
- Times of administration of each medication

Note: The MAR changes each day. Expired MARs are stored in the patients' charts.

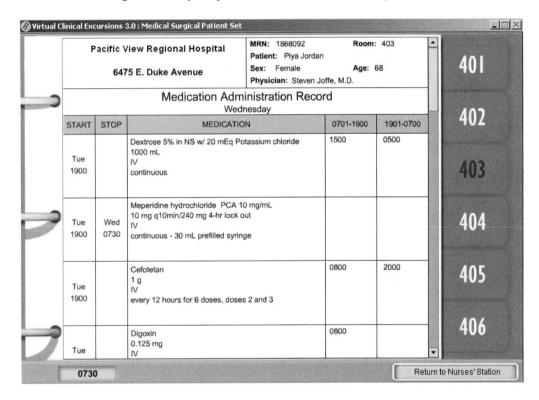

CHARTS

To access patient charts, either click on the **Chart** icon at the top of your screen or anywhere within the chart rack in the center of the Nurses' Station screen. When the close-up view appears, the individual charts are labeled by room number. To open a chart, click on the room number of the patient whose chart you wish to review. The patient's name and allergies will appear on the left side of the screen, along with a list of tabs on the right side of the screen, allowing you to view the following data:

- Allergies
- Physician's Orders
- Physician's Notes
- Nurse's Notes
- Laboratory Reports
- Diagnostic Reports
- Surgical Reports
- Consultations

- Patient Education
- History and Physical
- Nursing Admission
- Expired MARs
- Consents
- Mental Health
- Admissions
- Emergency Department

Information appears in real time. The entries are in reverse chronologic order, so use the down arrow at the right side of each chart page to scroll down to view previous entries. Flip from tab to tab to view multiple data fields or click on the **Return to Nurses' Station** bar in the lower right corner of the screen to exit the chart.

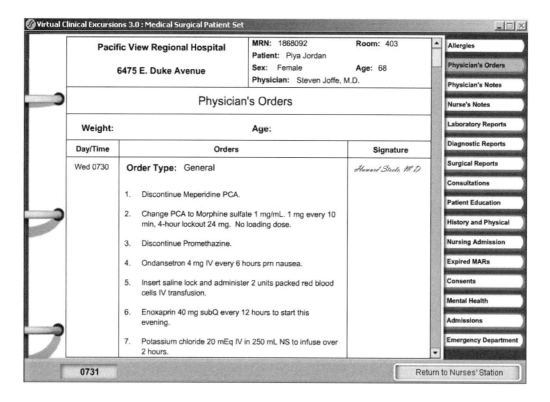

ELECTRONIC PATIENT RECORD (EPR)

The EPR can be accessed from the computer in the Nurses' Station or from the EPR icon located in the tool bar at the top of your screen. To access a patient's EPR:

- Click on either the computer screen or the **EPR** icon.
- Your username and password are automatically filled in.
- Click on **Login** to enter the EPR.
- *Note:* Like the MAR, the EPR is arranged numerically. Thus when you enter, you are initially shown the records of the patient in the lowest room number on the floor. To view the correct data for *your* patient, remember to select the correct room number, using the drop-down menu for the Patient field at the top left corner of the screen.

The EPR used in Pacific View Regional Hospital represents a composite of commercial versions being used in hospitals. You can access the EPR:

- to review existing data for a patient (by room number).
- to enter data you collect while working with a patient.

The EPR is updated daily, so no matter what day or part of a shift you are working, there will be a current EPR with the patient's data from the past days of the current hospital stay. This type of simulated EPR allows you to examine how data for different attributes have changed over time, as well as to examine data for all of a patient's attributes at a particular time. The EPR is fully functional (as it is in a real-life hospital). You can enter such data as blood pressure, breath sounds, and certain treatments. The EPR will not, however, allow you to enter data for a previous time period. Use the arrows at the bottom of the screen to move forward and backward in time.

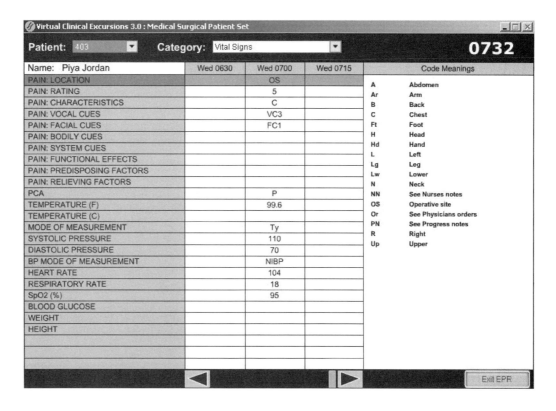

At the top of the EPR screen, you can choose patients by their room numbers. In addition, you have access to 17 different categories of patient data. To change patients or data categories, click the down arrow to the right of the room number or category.

The categories of patient data in the EPR as as follows:

- Vital Signs
- Respiratory
- Cardiovascular
- Neurologic
- Gastrointestinal
- Excretory
- Musculoskeletal
- Integumentary
- Reproductive
- Psychosocial
- Wounds and Drains
- Activity
- Hygiene and Comfort
- Safety
- Nutrition
- IV
- Intake and Output

Remember, each hospital selects its own codes. The codes used in the EPR at Pacific View Regional Hospital may be different from ones you have seen in your clinical rotations. Take some time to acquaint yourself with the codes. Within the Vital Signs category, click on any item in the left column (e.g., Pain: Characteristics). In the far-right column, you will see a list of code meanings for the possible findings and/or descriptors for that assessment area.

You will use the codes to record the data you collect as you work with patients. Click on the box in the last time column to the right of any item and wait for the code meanings applicable to that entry to appear. Select the appropriate code to describe your assessment findings and type it in the box. (*Note:* If no cursor appears within the box, click on the box again until the blue shading disappears and the blinking cursor appears.) Once the data are typed in this box, they are entered into the patient's record for this period of care only.

To leave the EPR, click on **Exit EPR** in the bottom right corner of the screen.

■ VISITING A PATIENT

From the Nurses' Station, click on the room number of the patient you wish to visit in the tool bar at the bottom of your screen. Once you are inside the room, you will see a still photo of your patient in the top left corner. To verify that this is the patient you have chosen, click on the **Check Armband** icon to the right of the photo. The patient's identification data will appear. If you click on **Check Allergies** (the next icon to the right), a list of the patient's allergies (if any) will replace the photo.

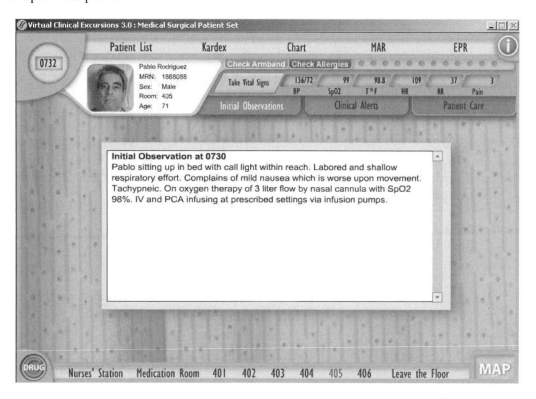

Also located in the patient's room are multiple icons you can use to assess the patient or the patient's medications. A virtual clock is provided in the upper left corner of the room to monitor your progress in real time. (*Note:* The fast-forward icon within the virtual clock will advance the time by 2-minute intervals when clicked.)

- The tool bar across the top of the screen allows you to check the **Patient List**, access the **EPR** to check or enter data, and view the patient's **Chart**, **MAR**, or **Kardex**.

- The **Take Vital Signs** icon allows you to measure the patient's up-to-the-minute blood pressure, oxygen saturation, temperature, heart rate, respiratory rate, and pain level.

- Each time you enter a patient's room, you are given an Initial Observation report to review (in the text box under the patient's photo). These notes are provided to give you a "look" at the patient as if you had just stepped into the room. You can also click on the **Initial Observations** icon to return to this box from other views within the patient's room. To the right of this icon is **Clinical Alerts**, a resource that allows you to make decisions about priority medication interventions based on emerging data collected in real time. Check this screen throughout your period of care to avoid missing critical information related to recently ordered or STAT medications.

- Clicking on the **Patient Care** icon opens up three specific learning environments within the patient room: **Physical Assessment**, **Nurse-Client Interactions**, and **Medication Administration**.

- To perform a **Physical Assessment**, choose a body area (such as **Head & Neck**) by clicking on the appropriate icon in the column of yellow buttons. This activates a list of system subcategories for that body area (e.g., see **Sensory**, **Neurologic**, etc. in the green boxes). After you click on the system that you wish to evaluate, a still photo and text box appear, describing the assessment findings. The still photo is a "snapshot" of how an assessment of this area might be done or what the finding might look like. For every body area, there is also an **Equipment** button located on the far right of the screen.

- To the right of the Physical Assessment icon is **Nurse-Client Interactions**. Clicking on this icon will reveal the times and titles of any videos available for viewing. (*Note:* If the video you wish to see is not listed, this means you have not yet reached the correct virtual time to view that video. Check the virtual clock; you may return to access the video once its designated time has occurred—as long as you do so within the same period of care. Or you can click on the fast-forward icon within the virtual clock to advance the time by 2-minute intervals. You will then need to click again on **Patient Care** and **Nurse-Client Interactions** to refresh the screen.) To view a listed video, click on the white arrow to the right of the video title. Use the control buttons below the video to start, stop, pause, rewind, or fast-forward the action or to mute the sound.

- **Medication Administration** is the pathway that allows you to review and administer medications to a patient after you have prepared them in the Medication Room. This process is addressed further in the *How to Prepare Medications* section (pages 19-20) and in *Medications* (pages 26-30). For additional hands-on practice, see *Reducing Medication Errors* (pages 37-41).

■ HOW TO QUIT, CHANGE PATIENTS, CHANGE FLOORS, OR CHANGE PERIOD OF CARE

How to Quit: From most screens, you may click the **Leave the Floor** icon on the bottom tool bar to the right of the patient room numbers. (*Note:* From some screens, you will first need to click an **Exit** button or **Return to Nurses' Station** before clicking **Leave the Floor**.) When the Floor Menu appears, click **Exit** to leave the program.

How to Change Patients, Floors, or Period of Care: To change patients, simply click on the new patient's room number. (You cannot receive a scorecard for a new patient, however, unless you have already selected that patient on the Patient List screen.) To change to a new period of care, to change floors, or to restart the virtual clock, click on **Leave the Floor** and then on **Restart the Program**.

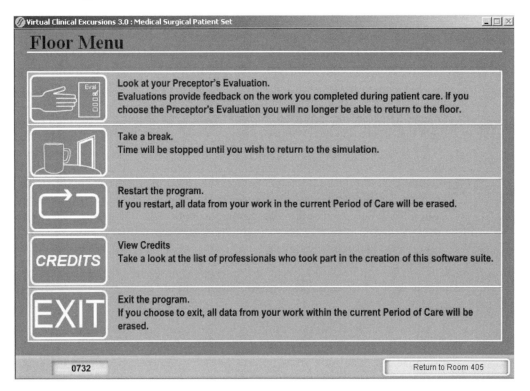

■ HOW TO PREPARE MEDICATIONS

From the Nurses' Station or the patient's room, you can access the Medication Room by clicking on the icon in the tool bar at the bottom of your screen to the left of the patient room numbers.

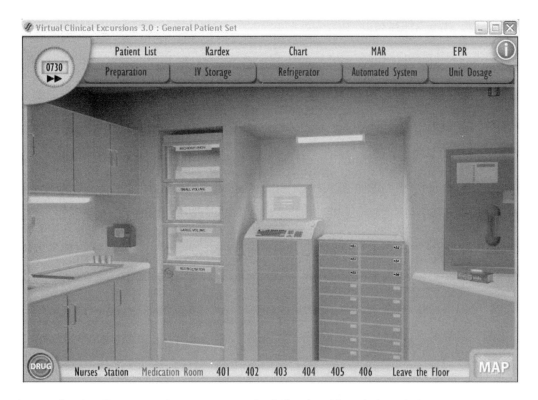

In the Medication Room you have access to the following (from left to right):

- A preparation area is located on the counter under the cabinets. To begin the medication preparation process, click on the tray on the counter or click on the **Preparation** icon at the top of the screen. The next screen leads you through a specific sequence (called the Preparation Wizard) to prepare medications one at a time for administration to a patient. However, no medication has been selected at this time. We will do this while working with a patient in *A Detailed Tour*. To exit this screen, click on **View Medication Room**.

- To the right of the cabinets (and above the refrigerator), IV storage bins are provided. Click on the bins themselves or on the **IV Storage** icon at the top of the screen. The bins are labeled **Microinfusion**, **Small Volume**, and **Large Volume**. Click on an individual bin to see a list of its contents. If you needed to prepare an IV medication at this time, you could click on the medication and its label would appear to the right under the patient's name. Next, you would click **Put Medication on Tray**. If you ever change your mind or choose the incorrect medication, you can reverse your actions by clicking on **Put Medication in Bin**. Click **Close Bin** in the right bottom corner to exit. **View Medication Room** brings you back to a full view of the entire room.

- A refrigerator is located under the IV storage bins to hold any medications that must be stored below room temperature. Click on the refrigerator door or on the **Refrigerator** icon at the top of the screen. Then click on the close-up view of the door to access the medications. When you are finished, click **Close Door** and then **View Medication Room**.

- To prepare controlled substances, click the **Automated System** icon at the top of the screen or click the computer monitor located to the right of the IV storage bins. A login screen will appear; your name and password are automatically filled in. Click **Login**. Select the patient for whom you wish to access medications; then select the correct medication drawer to open (they are stored alphabetically). Click **Open Drawer**, highlight the proper medication, and choose **Put Medication on Tray**. When you are finished, click **Close Drawer** and then **View Medication Room**.

- Next to the Automated System is a set of drawers identified by patient room number. To access these, click on the drawers themselves or on the **Unit Dosage** icon at the top of the screen. This provides a close-up view of the drawers. To open a drawer, click on the room number of the patient you are working with. Next, click on the medication you would like to prepare for the patient, and a label will appear to the right, listing the medication strength, units, and dosage per unit. You can **Open** and **Close** this medication label by clicking the appropriate icon. To exit, click **Close Drawer**; then click **View Medication Room**.

At any time, you can learn about a medication you wish to prepare for a patient by clicking on the **Drug** icon in the bottom left corner of the medication room screen or by clicking the **Drug Guide** book on the counter to the right of the unit dosage drawers. The **Drug Guide** provides information about the medications commonly included in nursing drug handbooks. Nutritional supplements and maintenance intravenous fluid preparations are not included.

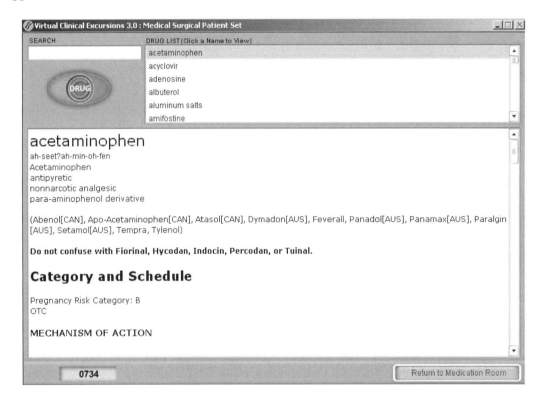

To access the MAR to review the medications ordered for a patient, click on the **MAR** icon located in the tool bar at the top of your screen and then click on the correct tab for your patient's room number. You may also click the **Review MAR** icon in the tool bar at the bottom of your screen from inside each medication storage area.

After you have chosen and prepared your medications, return to the patient's room to administer them by clicking on the room number in the bottom tool bar. Once inside the patient's room, click on **Patient Care** and then on **Medication Administration** and follow the proper administration sequence.

■ PRECEPTOR'S EVALUATIONS

When you have finished a session, click on **Leave the Floor** to go to the Floor Menu. At this point, you can click on the top icon (**Look at Your Preceptor's Evaluation**) to receive a score-card that provides feedback on the work you completed during patient care.

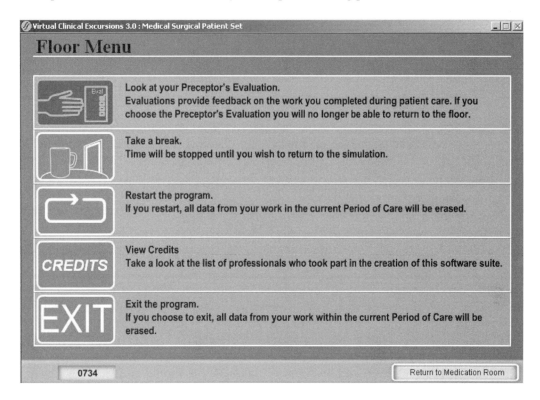

Evaluations are available for each patient you selected when you signed in for the current period of care. Click on the **Medication Scorecard** icon to see an example.

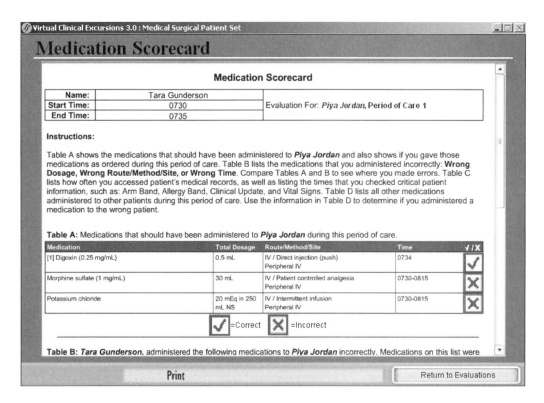

The scorecard compares the medications you administered to a patient during a period of care with what should have been administered. Table A lists the correct medications. Table B lists any medications that were administered incorrectly.

Remember, not every medication listed on the MAR should necessarily be given. For example, a patient might have an allergy to a drug that was ordered, or a medication might have been improperly transcribed to the MAR. Predetermined medication "errors" embedded within the program challenge you to exercise critical thinking skills and professional judgment when deciding to administer a medication, just as you would in a real hospital. Use all your available resources, such as the patient's chart and the MAR, to make your decision.

Table C lists the resources that were available to assist you in medication administration. It also documents whether and when you accessed these resources. For example, did you check the patient armband or perform a check of vital signs? If so, when?

You can click **Print** to get a copy of this report if needed. When you have finished reviewing the scorecard, click **Return to Evaluations** and then **Return to Menu**.

■ FLOOR MAP

To get a general sense of your location within the hospital, you can click on the **Map** icon found in the lower right corner of most of the screens in the *Virtual Clinical Excursions—General Hospital* program. (*Note:* If you are following this quick tour step by step, you will need to **Restart the Program** from the Floor Menu, sign in again, and go to the Nurses' Station to access the map.) When you click the **Map** icon, a floor map appears, showing the layout of the floor you are currently on, as well as a directory of the patients and services on that floor. As you move your cursor over the directory list, the location of each room is highlighted on the map (and vice versa). The floor map can be accessed from the Nurses' Station, Medication Room, and each patient's room.

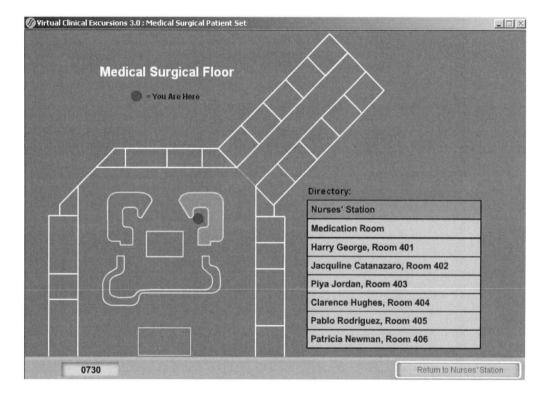

A DETAILED TOUR

If you wish to more thoroughly understand the capabilities of *Virtual Clinical Excursions—General Hospital*, take a detailed tour by completing the following section. During this tour, we will work with a specific patient to introduce you to all the different components and learning opportunities available within the software.

■ WORKING WITH A PATIENT

Sign in and select the Medical-Surgical floor for Period of Care 1 (0730-0815). From the Patient List, select Piya Jordan and Pablo Rodriguez; however, do not go to the Nurses' Station yet.

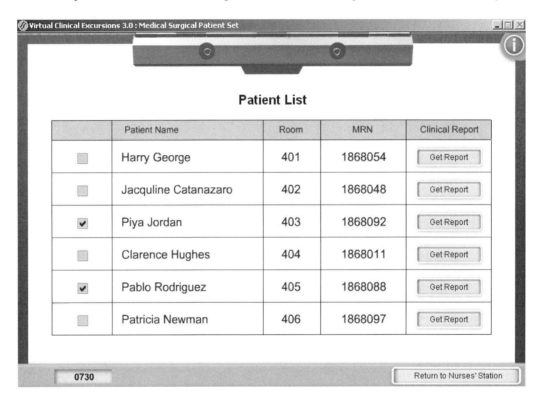

■ REPORT

In hospitals, when one shift ends and another begins, the outgoing nurse who attended a patient will give a verbal and sometimes a written summary of that patient's condition to the incoming nurse who will assume care for the patient. This summary is called a report and is an important source of data to provide an overview of a patient. Your first task is to get the clinical report on Piya Jordan. To do this, click **Get Report** in the far right column in this patient's row. From a brief review of this summary, identify the problems and areas of concern that you will need to address for this patient.

When you have finished noting any areas of concern, click on **Go to Nurses' Station**.

■ CHARTS

You can access Piya Jordan's chart from the Nurses' Station or from the patient's room (403). We will access it from the Nurses' Station: Click on the chart rack or on the **Chart** icon in the tool bar at the top of your screen. Next, click on the chart labeled **403** to open the medical record for Piya Jordan. Click on the **Emergency Department** tab to view a record of why this patient was admitted.

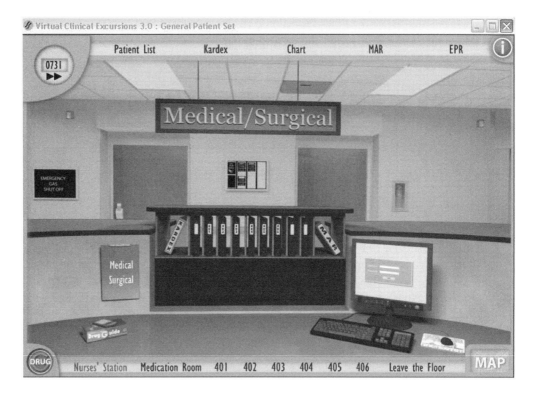

How many days has Piya Jordan been in the hospital?

What tests were done upon her arrival in the Emergency Department and why?

What was her reason for admission?

You should also click on **Surgical Reports** to learn what procedures were performed and when. Finally, review the **Nursing Admission** and **History and Physical** to learn about the health history of this patient. When you are done reviewing the chart, click **Return to Nurses' Station**.

■ MEDICATIONS

Open the Medication Administration Record (MAR) by clicking on the **MAR** icon in the tool bar at the top of your screen. *Remember:* The MAR automatically opens to the first occupied room number on the floor—which is not necessarily your patient's room number! Since you need to access Piya Jordan's MAR, click on tab **403** (her room number). Always make sure you are giving the *Right Drug to the Right Patient!*

Examine the list of medications ordered for Piya Jordan. In the table below, list the medications that need to be given during this period of care (0730-0815). For each medication, note the dosage, route, and time to be given.

Time	Medication	Dosage	Route

Click on **Return to Nurses' Station**. Next, click on **403** on the bottom tool bar and then verify that you are indeed in Piya Jordan's room. Select **Clinical Alerts** (the icon to the right of Initial Observations) to check for any emerging data that might affect your medication administration priorities. Next, go to the patient's chart (click on the **Chart** icon; then click on **403**). When the chart opens, select the **Physician's Orders** tab.

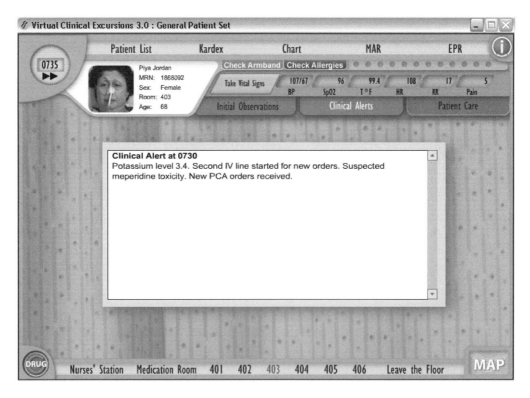

Review the orders. Have any new medications been ordered? Return to the MAR (click **Return to Room 403**; then click **MAR**). Verify that the new medications have been correctly transcribed to the MAR. Mistakes are sometimes made in the transcription process in the hospital setting, and it is sound practice to double-check any new order.

Are there any patient assessments you will need to perform before administering these medications? If so, return to Room 403 and click on **Patient Care** and then **Physical Assessment** to complete those assessments before proceeding.

Now click on the **Medication Room** icon in the tool bar at the bottom of your screen to locate and prepare the medications for Piya Jordan.

In the Medication Room, you must access the medications for Piya Jordan from the specific dispensing system in which each medication is stored. Locate each medication that needs to be given in this time period and click on **Put Medication on Tray** as appropriate. (*Hint:* Look in Unit Dosage drawer first.) When you are finished, click on **Close Drawer** and then on **View Medication Room**. Now click on the medication tray on the counter on the left side of the medication room screen to begin preparing the medications you have selected. (*Remember:* You can also click **Preparation** in the tool bar at the top of the screen.)

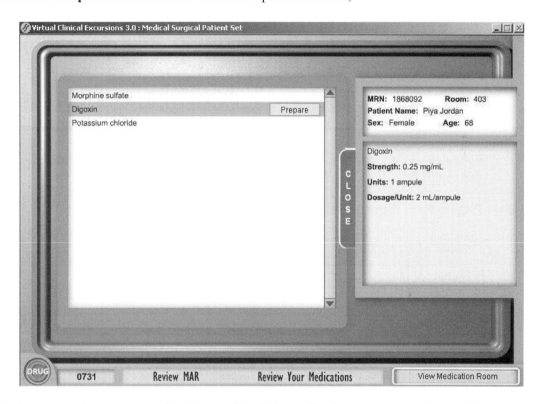

In the preparation area, you should see a list of the medications you put on the tray in the previous steps. Click on the first medication and then click **Prepare**. Follow the onscreen instructions of the Preparation Wizard, providing any data requested. As an example, let's follow the preparation process for digoxin, one of the medications due to be administered to Piya Jordan during this period of care. To begin, click to select **Digoxin**; then click **Prepare**. Now work through the Preparation Wizard sequence as detailed below:

Amount of medication in the ampule: 2 mL.
Enter the amount of medication you will draw up into a syringe: **0.5** mL.
Click **Next**.
Select the patient you wish to set aside the medication for: **Room 403, Piya Jordan**.
Click **Finish**.
Click **Return to Medication Room**.

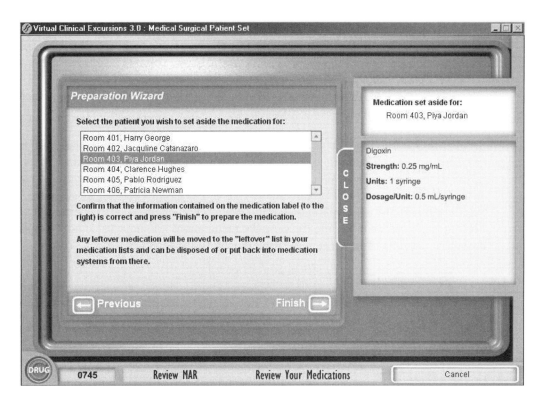

Follow this same basic process for the other medications due to be administered to Piya Jordan during this period of care. (*Hint:* Look in **IV Storage** and **Automated System**.)

PREPARATION WIZARD EXCEPTIONS

- Some medications in *Virtual Clinical Excursions—General Hospital* are prepared by the pharmacy (e.g., IV antibiotics) and taken to the patient room as a whole. This is common practice in most hospitals.
- Blood products are not administered by students through the *Virtual Clinical Excursions— General Hospital* simulations since blood administration follows specific protocols not covered in this program.
- The *Virtual Clinical Excursions—General Hospital* simulations do not allow for mixing more than one type of medication, such as regular and Lente insulins, in the same syringe. In the clinical setting, when multiple types of insulin are ordered for a patient, the regular insulin is drawn up first, followed by the longer-acting insulin. Insulin is always administered in a special unit-marked syringe.

Now return to Room 403 (click on **403** on the bottom tool bar) to administer Piya Jordan's medications.

At any time during the medication administration process, you can perform a further review of systems, take vital signs, check information contained within the chart, or verify patient identity and allergies. Inside Piya Jordan's room, click **Take Vital Signs**. (*Note:* These findings change over time to reflect the temporal changes you would find in a patient similar to Piya Jordan.)

When you have gathered all the data you need, click on **Patient Care** and then select **Medication Administration**. Any medications you prepared in the previous steps should be listed on the left side of your screen. Let's continue the administration process with the digoxin ordered for Piya Jordan. Click to highlight **Digoxin** in the list of medications. Next, click on the down arrow to the right of **Select** and choose **Administer** from the drop-down menu. This will activate the Administration Wizard. Complete the Wizard sequence as follows:

- Route: **IV**
- Method: **Direct Injection**
- Site: **Peripheral IV**
- Click **Administer to Patient** arrow.
- Would you like to document this administration in the MAR? **Yes**
- Click **Finish** arrow.

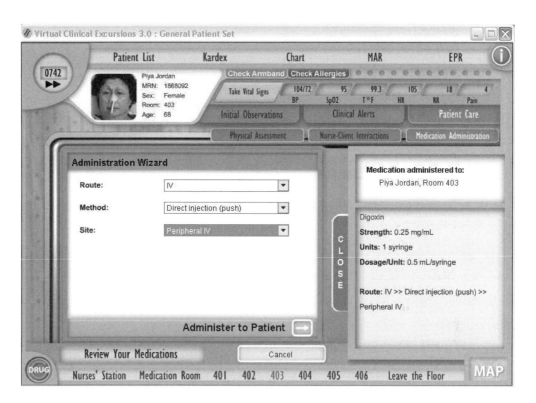

Your selections are recorded by a tracking system and evaluated on a Medication Scorecard stored under Preceptor's Evaluations. This scorecard can be viewed, printed, and given to your instructor. To access the Preceptor's Evaluations, click on **Leave the Floor**. When the Floor Menu appears, click on the icon next to **Look at Your Preceptor's Evaluation**. Then click on **Medication Scorecard** inside the box with Piya Jordan's name (see example on the following page).

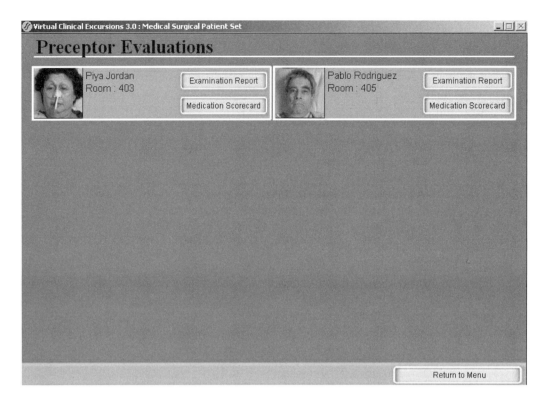

■ MEDICATION SCORECARD

- First, review Table A. Was digoxin given correctly? Did you give the other medications as ordered?
- Table B shows you which (if any) medications you gave incorrectly.
- Table C addresses the resources used for Piya Jordan. Did you access the patient's chart, MAR, EPR, or Kardex as needed to make safe medication administration decisions?
- Did you check the patient's armband to verify her identity? Did you check whether your patient had any known allergies to medications? Were vital signs taken?

When you have finished reviewing the scorecard, click **Return to Evaluations** and then **Return to Menu**.

■ VITAL SIGNS

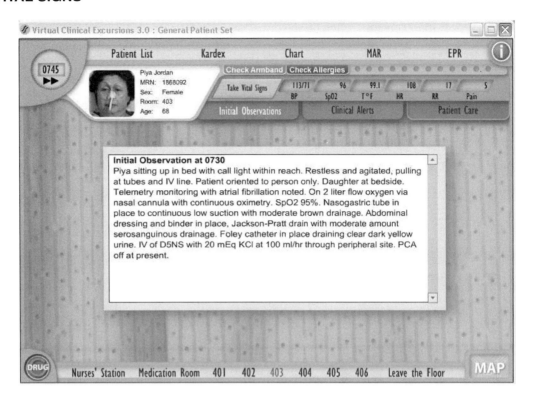

Vital signs, often considered the traditional "signs of life," include body temperature, heart rate, respiratory rate, blood pressure, oxygen saturation of the blood, and pain level.

Inside Piya Jordan's room, click **Take Vital Signs**. (*Note:* If you are following this detailed tour step by step, you will need to **Restart the Program** from the Floor Menu, sign in again, and navigate to Room 403.) Collect vital signs for this patient and record them in the following table. Note the time at which you collected each of these data. (*Remember:* You can take vital signs at any time. The data change over time to reflect the temporal changes you would find in a patient similar to Piya Jordan.)

Vital Signs	Findings/Time
Blood pressure	
O$_2$ saturation	
Heart rate	
Respiratory rate	
Temperature	
Pain rating	

After you are done, click on the **EPR** icon located in the tool bar at the top of the screen. Your username and password are automatically provided. Click on **Login** to enter the EPR. To access Piya Jordan's records, click on the down arrow next to Patient and choose her room number, **403**. Select **Vital Signs** as the category. Next, in the empty time column on the far right, record the vital signs data you just collected in Piya Jordan's room. (*Note:* If you need help with this process, see page 16.) Now compare these findings with the data you collected earlier for this patient's vital signs. Use these earlier findings to establish a baseline for each of the vital signs.

    a. Are any of the data you collected significantly different from the baseline for a particular vital sign?

       Circle One: Yes   No

    b. If "Yes," which data are different?

■ PHYSICAL ASSESSMENT

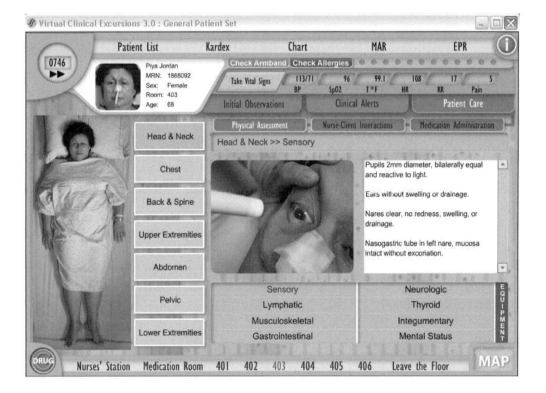

After you have finished examining the EPR for vital signs, click **Exit EPR** to return to Room 403. Click **Patient Care** and then **Physical Assessment**. Think about what information you received in the report at the beginning of this shift, as well as what you may have learned about this patient from the chart. Based on this, what area(s) of examination should you pay most attention to at this time? Is there any equipment you should be monitoring? Conduct a physical assessment of the body areas and systems that you consider priorities for Piya Jordan. For example, select **Head & Neck**; then click on and assess **Sensory** and **Lymphatic**. Complete any other assessment(s) you think are necessary at this time. In the following table, record the data you collected during this examination.

Area of Examination	Findings
Head & Neck Sensory	
Head & Neck Lymphatic	

After you have finished collecting these data, return to the EPR. Compare the data that were already in the record with those you just collected.

    a.   Are any of the data you collected significantly different from the baselines for this patient?

       Circle One: Yes   No

    b.   If "Yes," which data are different?

■ **NURSE-CLIENT INTERACTIONS**

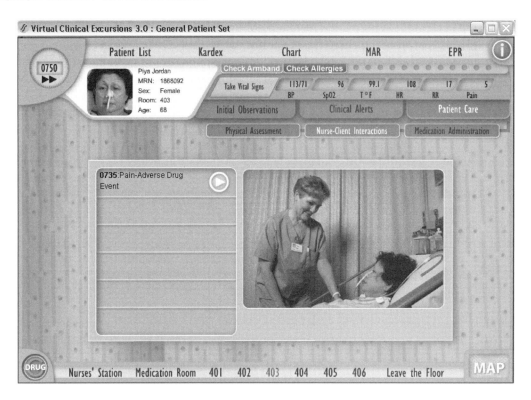

Click on **Patient Care** from inside Piya Jordan's room (403). Now click on **Nurse-Client Interactions** to access a short video titled **Pain—Adverse Drug Event**, which is available for viewing at or after 0735 (based on the virtual clock in the upper left corner of your screen; see *Note* below). To begin the video, click on the arrow next to its title. You will observe a nurse communicating with Piya Jordan and her daughter. There are many variations of nursing practice, some exemplifying "best" practice and some not. Note whether the nurse in this interaction displays professional behavior and compassionate care. Are her words congruent with what is going on with the patient? Does this interaction "feel right" to you? If not, how would you handle this situation differently? Explain.

Note: If the video you wish to view is not listed, this means you have not yet reached the correct virtual time to view that video. Check the virtual clock; you may return to access the video once its designated time has occurred—as long as you do so within the same period of care. Or you can click on the fast-forward icon within the virtual clock to advance the time by 2-minute intervals. You will then need to click again on **Patient Care** and **Nurse-Client Interactions** to refresh the screen.

At least one Nurse-Client Interactions video is available during each period of care. Viewing these videos can help you learn more about what is occurring with a patient at a certain time and also prompt you to discern between nurse communications that are ideal and those that need improvement. Compassionate care and the ability to communicate clearly are essential components of delivering quality nursing care, and it is during your clinical time that you will begin to refine these skills.

■ COLLECTING AND EVALUATING DATA

Each of the activities you perform in the Patient Care environment generates a significant amount of assessment data. Remember that after you collect data, you can record your findings in the EPR. You can also review the EPR, patient's chart, videos, and MAR at any time. You will get plenty of practice collecting and then evaluating data in context of the patient's course.

Now, here's an important question for you:

> Did the previous sequence of exercises provide the most efficient way to assess Piya Jordan?

For example, you went to the patient's room to get vital signs, then back to the EPR to enter data and compare your findings with extant data. Next, you went back to the patient's room to do a physical examination, then again back to the EPR to enter and review data. If this back-and-forth process of data collection and recording seemed inefficient, remember the following:

- Plan all of your nursing activities to maximize efficiency, while at the same time optimizing the quality of patient care. (Think about what data you might need before performing certain tasks. For example, do you need to check a heart rate before administering a cardiac medication or check an IV site before starting an infusion?)

- You collect a tremendous amount of data when you work with a patient. Very few people can accurately remember all these data for more than a few minutes. Develop efficient assessment skills, and record data as soon as possible after collecting them.

- Assessment data are only the starting point for the nursing process.

Make a clear distinction between these first exercises and how you actually provide nursing care. These initial exercises were designed to involve you actively in the use of different software components. This workbook focuses on sensible practices for implementing the nursing process in ways that ensure the highest-quality care of patients.

Most important, remember that a human being changes through time, and that these changes include both the physical and psychosocial facets of a person as a living organism. Think about this for a moment. Some patients may change physically in a very short time (a patient with emerging myocardial infarction) or more slowly (a patient with a chronic illness). Patients' overall physical and psychosocial conditions may improve or deteriorate. They may have effective coping skills and familial support, or they may feel alone and full of despair. In fact, each individual is a complex mix of physical and psychosocial elements, and at least some of these elements usually change through time.

Thus it is crucial that you *DO NOT* think of the nursing process as a simple one-time, five-step procedure consisting of assessment, nursing diagnosis, planning, implementation, and evaluation. Rather, the nursing process should be utilized as a creative and systematic approach to delivering nursing care. Furthermore, because all living organisms are constantly changing, we must apply the nursing process over and over. Each time we follow the nursing process for an individual patient, we refine our understanding of that patient's physical and psychosocial conditions based on collection and analysis of many different types of data. *Virtual Clinical Excursions—General Hospital* will help you develop both the creativity and the systematic approach needed to become a nurse who is equipped to deliver the highest-quality care to all patients.

REDUCING MEDICATION ERRORS

Earlier in this detailed tour, you learned the basic steps of medication preparation and administration. The following simulations will allow you to practice those skills further—with an increased emphasis on reducing medication errors by using the Medication Scorecard to evaluate your work.

Sign in to work at Pacific View Regional Hospital for Period of Care 1. (*Note:* If you are already working with another patient or during another period of care, click on **Leave the Floor** and then **Restart the Program**; then sign in.)

From the Patient List, select Clarence Hughes. Then click on **Go to Nurses' Station**. Complete the following steps to prepare and administer medications to Clarence Hughes.

- Click on **Medication Room**.
- Click on **MAR** and then on tab **404** to determine prn medications that have been ordered for Clarence Hughes to address his constipation and pain. (*Note:* You may click on **Review MAR** at any time to verify the correct medication order. Always remember to check the patient name on the MAR to make sure you have the correct patient's record—you must click on the correct room number tab within the MAR.) Click on **Return to Medication Room** after reviewing the correct MAR.
- Click on **Unit Dosage** (or on the Unit Dosage cabinet); from the close-up view, click on drawer **404**.
- Select the medications you would like to administer. After each selection, click **Put Medication on Tray**. When you are finished selecting medications, click **Close Drawer** and then **View Medication Room**.
- Click **Automated System** (or on the Automated System unit itself). Click **Login**.
- On the next screen, specify the correct patient and drawer location.
- Select the medication you would like to administer and click **Put Medication on Tray**. Repeat this process if you wish to administer other medications from the Automated System.
- When you are finished, click **Close Drawer** and **View Medication Room**.
- From the Medication Room, click **Preparation** (or on the preparation tray).
- From the list of medications on your tray, highlight the correct medication to administer and click **Prepare**.
- This activates the Preparation Wizard. Supply any requested information; then click **Next**.
- Now select the correct patient to receive this medication and click **Finish**.
- Repeat the previous three steps until all medications that you want to administer are prepared.
- You can click on **Review Your Medications** and then on **Return to Medication Room** when ready. Once you are back in the Medication Room, go directly to Clarence Hughes' room by clicking on **404** at the bottom of the screen.
- Inside the patient's room, administer the medication, utilizing the five rights of medication administration. After you have collected the appropriate assessment data and are ready for administration, click **Patient Care** and then **Medication Administration**. Verify that the correct patient and medication(s) appear in the left-hand window. Highlight the first medication you wish to administer; then click the down arrow next to Select. From the drop-down menu, select **Administer** and complete the Administration Wizard by providing any information requested. When the Wizard stops asking for information, click **Administer to Patient**. Specify **Yes** when asked whether this administration should be recorded in the MAR. Finally, click **Finish**.

■ **SELF-EVALUATION**

Now let's see how you did during your medication administration!

• Click on **Leave the Floor** at the bottom of your screen. From the Floor Menu, select **Look at Your Preceptor's Evaluation**. Then click **Medication Scorecard**.

These resources will help you find out more about each patient's medications and possible sources of medication errors.

1. Start by examining Table A. These are the medications you should have given to Clarence Hughes during this period of care. If each of the medications in Table A has a ✓ by it, then you made no errors. Congratulations!

If any medication has an X by it, then you made one or more medication errors.

Compare Tables A and B to determine which of the following types of errors you made: Wrong Dose, Wrong Route/Method/Site, or Wrong Time. Follow these steps:

a. Find medications in Table A that were given incorrectly.
b. Now see if those same medications are in Table B, which shows what you actually administered to Clarence Hughes.
c. Comparing Tables A and B, match the Strength, Dose, Route/Method/Site, and Time for each medication you administered incorrectly.
d. Then, using the form below, list the medications given incorrectly and mark the errors you made for each medication.

Medication	Strength	Dosage	Route	Method	Site	Time
	❑	❑	❑	❑	❑	❑
	❑	❑	❑	❑	❑	❑
	❑	❑	❑	❑	❑	❑
	❑	❑	❑	❑	❑	❑

2. To help you reduce future medication errors, consider the following list of possible reasons for errors.

• Did not check drug against MAR for correct patient, correct date, correct time, correct drug, and correct dose.
• Did not check drug dose against MAR three times.
• Did not open the unit dose package in the patient's room.
• Did not correctly identify the patient using two identifiers.
• Did not administer the drug on time.
• Did not verify patient allergies.
• Did not check the patient's current condition or vital sign parameters.
• Did not consider why the patient would be receiving this drug.
• Did not question why the drug was in the patient's drawer.
• Did not check the physician's order and/or check with the pharmacist when there was a question about the drug or dose.
• Did not verify that no adverse effects had occurred from a previous dose.

Based on these possibilities, determine how you made each error and record the reason into the form below:

Medication	Reason for Error

3. Look again at Table B. Are there medications listed that are not in Table A? If so, you gave a medication to Clarence Hughes that he should not have received. Complete the following exercises to help you understand how such an error might have been made.

   a. Perhaps you gave a medication that was on Clarence Hughes' MAR for this period of care, without recognizing that a change had occurred in the patient's condition, which should have caused you to reconsider. Review patient records as necessary and complete the following form:

Medication	Possible Reasons Not to Give This Medication

   b. Another possibility is that you gave Clarence Hughes a medication that should have been given at a different time. Check his MAR and complete the form below to determine whether you made a Wrong Time error:

Medication	Given to Clarence Hughes at What Time	Should Have Been Given at What Time

c. Maybe you gave another patient's medication to Clarence Hughes. In this case, you made a Wrong Patient error. Check the MARs of other patients and use the form below to determine whether you made this type of error:

Medication	Given to Clarence Hughes	Should Have Been Given to

4. The Medication Scorecard provides some other interesting sources of information. For example, if there is a medication selected for Clarence Hughes but it was not given to him, there will be an X by that medication in Table A, but it will not appear in Table B. In that case, you might have given this medication to some other patient, which is another type of Wrong Patient error. To investigate further, look at Table D, which lists the medications you gave to other patients. See whether you can find any medications for Clarence Hughes that were given to another patient by mistake. However, before you make any decisions, be sure to cross-check the MAR for other patients because the same medication may have been ordered for multiple patients. Use the following form to record your findings:

Medication	Should Have Been Given to Clarence Hughes	Given by Mistake to

5. Now take some time to review the medication exercises you just completed. Use the form below to create an overall analysis of what you have learned. Once again, record each of the medication errors you made, including the type of each error. Then, for each error you made, indicate specifically what you would do differently to prevent this type of error from occurring again.

Medication	Type of Error	Error Prevention Tactic

Submit this form to your instructor if required as a graded assignment, or simply use these exercises to improve your understanding of medication errors and how to reduce them.

Name: _____   Date: _____

The following icons are used throughout the workbook to help you quickly identify particular activities and assignments:

 Indicates a reading assignment—tells you which textbook chapter(s) you should read before starting each lesson

 Indicates a writing activity

 Marks the beginning of an interactive CD-ROM activity—signals you to open or return to your *Virtual Clinical Excursions—General Hospital* CD-ROM

 Indicates additional CD-ROM instructions

 Indicates questions and activities that require you to consult your textbook

 Indicates the approximate time required to complete an exercise

LESSON 1

Ethics and Nursing Care

⚯ **Reading Assignment:** Ethical and Legal Context of Practice (Chapter 2)

Client: Goro Oishi, Skilled Nursing Floor, Room 505

Objectives:

1. Apply ethical principles to clarify values and make decisions in nursing.
2. Define key terms associated with ethical and legal elements in nursing practice.
3. Identify the steps used in the resolution of a moral dilemma.
4. Identify the elements of the codes of ethics for nursing.

Exercise 1

Writing Activity

30 minutes

1. When providing care to clients, the nurse is faced with both ethical and legal concerns. Knowledge and understanding of the scope of practice and appropriate steps to take are necessary for safe, effective practice. Match each of the key terms below with its correct definition.

Key Terms	**Definition**
_____ Values	a. Examines the behavior to determine what will constitute good, bad, right, and wrong
_____ Morals	b. Adherence to the truth
_____ Ethics	c. The right to make individual choices
_____ Autonomy	d. Honoring agreements and keeping promises
_____ Beneficence	e. Ideals, beliefs, and patterns of behaviors
_____ Nonmaleficence	f. Moral rightness, fairness, or equality
_____ Fidelity	g. Standards of conduct that represent the ideal of human behavior
_____ Justice	h. The promotion of good
_____ Veracity	i. Implies that the good of actions should outweigh any possible harm to clients

2. A client presents with issues that give rise to a moral dilemma. Put the following steps for resolving the ethical dilemma in order of priority.

_____ Clarifying viewpoints of individuals involved	a. First
_____ Selection of action and examination of possible outcomes related to the action	b. Second
_____ Recognition of a moral situation	c. Third
_____ Intention to implement morally correct behavior	d. Fourth
_____ Examination of possible courses of action	e. Fifth
_____ Performance of a selected behavior	f. Sixth

3. When a person understands what actions should be taken but support is lacking to assist in reaching a final decision or implementation of an action, _____ results.

4. _____ refers to the situation that results when a person is unsure whether a true moral or ethical dilemma exists.

5. According to the International Council of Nurses (ICN) Code of Ethics for Nurses, there are four principal elements that outline the standards of ethical conduct. List these elements.

6. A nurse has intentionally documented inaccurate medication administration information in the client's permanent record. This is an example of:
   a. Defamation
   b. Assault
   c. A tort
   d. Fraud

Exercise 2

 CD-ROM Activity

 30 minutes

- Sign in to work at Pacific View Regional Hospital on the Skilled Nursing Floor for Period of Care 2. (*Note:* If you are already in the virtual hospital from a previous exercise, click on **Leave the Floor** and then **Restart the Program** to get to the sign-in window.)
- From the Patient List, select Goro Oishi (Room 505).
- Click on **Get Report** and read the report.
- Click on **Go to Nurses' Station** and then on **505** at the bottom of the screen.
- Review the **Initial Observations**.
- Next, click on **Chart** and then on **505**.
- Click on and review the **Physician's Orders**, **Physician's Notes**, and **History and Physical** sections.

1. What are Goro Oishi's two admitting diagnoses?

2. What has been identified as the plan of action concerning Goro Oishi's condition?

A review of the chart's contents reveals that not all members of Goro Oishi's family are in agreement concerning the plan of care. There are times in nursing practice when a nurse will face conflicts between personal beliefs and values and the plan of care being implemented.

3. What potential dilemmas regarding the plan of care for Goro Oishi may exist for the nurse assigned to provide care?

 The Jameton Model provides a six-step process to assist in ethical decision making. Use the components of this model to respond to the potential issues and concerns regarding the Do Not Resuscitate plan for Goro Oishi posed in the following questions. Consider the conflicts between his family members and possibly the nurse's own belief system. (*Hint:* See page 22 in your textbook.)

4. **Step 1: Identify the Ethical Dilemma.**
   What is the ethical problem in Goro Oishi's situation? Is it a matter of ethics, a legal issue, or a question of communication? Are there ethical principles in conflict?

5. **Step 2: Gather Pertinent Data.**
   Who are the people involved? Is there a conflict of values? Are there cultural influences? What are the financial implications?

6. **Step 3: Examine the Dilemma for Ethical Principles.**
   Have all of the principal parties been given the necessary information? Whose interests are being served?

7. **Step 4: Examine All Solutions.**
   What options are open to the family?

8. **Step 5: Choose Solutions.**
   Are available and selected solutions consistent with ethical principles?

9. **Step 6: Evaluate Solutions Chosen.**
   After the decision has been implemented, questions can be used to reflect on the effectiveness of the plan selected in resolving the ethical dilemma. Were additional issues identified during the process?

LESSON 2

Culture and Nursing Practice

Reading Assignment: Cultural Context of Practice (Chapter 3)

Clients: William Jefferson, Skilled Nursing Floor, Room 501
Goro Oishi, Skilled Nursing Floor, Room 505

Objectives:

1. Discuss culture and ethnicity as they relate to the delivery of nursing care.
2. Define humanistic care.
3. Outline the elements and objectives of transcultural nursing.
4. List and explain the six concepts included in transcultural assessment.
5. Anticipate the effects of cultural characteristics on the successful delivery of health care.

Exercise 1

Clinical Preparation: Writing Activity

30 minutes

1. Culture is defined as patterned behavioral responses that develop over time. What factors work together to shape culture?

Copyright © 2007 by Saunders, an imprint of Elsevier Inc. All rights reserved.

2. When identifying the traits of an ethnic group, the nurse may consider which of the following primary characteristics? Select all that apply.

   _____   Race

   _____   Color

   _____   Health care practices

   _____   Moral values

   _____   Language

   _____   Cultural origin

   _____   National or geographical origin

3. What secondary characteristics should be given consideration when identifying ethnic groups? Select all that apply.

   _____   A sense of group identity

   _____   Cultural origin

   _____   Attitudes derived from group identity

   _____   Distinctive customs, art, music, literature

   _____   Elements of lifestyles

   _____   Food preferences

4. Care that includes understanding and knowledge of a client in a natural or human way is

   known as _____.

5. An individual's opinion that his or her own religious choices are best and superior to those practiced by different groups demonstrates which of the following concepts?
   a. Monoculturalism
   b. Ethnocentrism
   c. Stereotyping
   d. Biculturalism

6. A nurse caring for an infant of Chinese descent should be aware of the high incidence of jaundice.
   a. True
   b. False

7. Chinese Americans may be more susceptible to which of the following diet-related disorders and diseases?

_____ Heart disease

_____ Cancer of the bowel

_____ Breast cancer

_____ Stomach cancer

_____ Lactose intolerance

_____ Thalassemia deficiency

8. Which of the following cultures traditionally believes that touching a dead person is taboo?
   a. Japanese
   b. Chinese
   c. Navajo
   d. African

9. What is cultural competence?

10. List the seven elements and skills associated with cultural competence.

Exercise 2

 CD-ROM Activity

 30 minutes

- Sign in to work at Pacific View Regional Hospital on the Skilled Nursing Floor for Period of Care 1. (*Note:* If you are already in the virtual hospital from a previous exercise, click on **Leave the Floor** and then **Restart the Program** to get to the sign-in window.)
- From the Patient List, select William Jefferson (Room 501) and Goro Oishi (Room 505).
- Click on **Get Report** and read the reports for each of the clients.
- Click on **Go to Nurses' Station**.
- Click on **501** at the bottom of the screen and review the **Initial Observations**.
- Click on **Chart** and then on **501**.
- Click on and review the **History and Physical** and Nursing Admission tabs.

1. Identify the ethnic group to which William Jefferson belongs.

2. How do the meanings of the terms *black* and *African-American* differ?

3. According to the History and Physical in William Jefferson's chart, what cultural and community activities are of high priority in his family?

4. Are the Jefferson family's social priorities similar to those historically held in high esteem by the African-American community? Why or why not?

5. The Jefferson family reflects a _____, or male-headed, family unit.

6. When providing care to William Jefferson, the nurse must be knowledgeable of health conditions for which he is at higher risk because of his ethnic/racial background. Which of the following diseases/disorders does William Jefferson have an increased risk for developing?

_____ Diabetes

_____ Lactose intolerance

_____ Hypertension

_____ Osteoporosis

_____ Cardiovascular disease

_____ Cirrhosis

_____ Sickle cell disease

→ • Click on **Return to Room 501**.
  • Now click on **505** to go to Goro Oishi's room.
  • Review the **Initial Observations**.
  • Click on **Chart** and then on **505**.
  • Click on and review the **History and Physical** and **Nursing Admission** tabs.

7. Identify the ethnic group to which Goro Oishi belongs.

8. Discuss three traditional values/behaviors of Asian-Americans.

9. What behaviors characteristic of Asian-Americans did Goro Oishi exhibit prior to his collapse? (*Hint:* See the Social History within the History and Physical.)

10. What behaviors reportedly displayed by Goro Oishi's wife are characteristic of Asian-Americans? (*Hint:* See the Social History within the History and Physical.)

11. In traditional Asian-American families, the elders are respected and revered. Is this system of familial hierarchy supported by the Oishi family?

LESSON **3**

The Client Assessment

/OR̃O **Reading Assignment:** Client Assessment: Nursing History (Chapter 6)
Physical Assessment (Chapter 8)

Client: William Jefferson, Skilled Nursing Floor, Room 501

Objectives:

1. Use effective interviewing techniques in taking a health history.
2. Describe the four techniques used in physical examination.
3. Identify the purpose of the primary instruments used in physical assessment.
4. Perform a complete physical examination on a client using a head-to-toe approach.
5. Recognize normal physical findings.
6. Recognize when physical findings that deviate from normal.

Exercise 1

Writing Activity

30 minutes

1. Match each of the following types of assessment with its correct definition.

Assessment Type	Definition
Focused	a. An assessment including only key data related to the immediate problem
b. Initial	b. An assessment performed when the client and nurse interaction first begins
c Emergency	c. A detailed assessment of a specific problem
d Ongoing	d. Continuous or episodic assessment

2. A client reports experiencing pain and tenderness in the shoulder. These reports are examples of objective data.
   a. True
   b. False *(circled)*

3. _active_ processing uses systematic mental actions to analyze and interpret information about the client.

4. The client reports recent symptoms to the nurse. During the data collection, the nurse believes she has an idea about what is troubling the client. The behavior being exhibited by the nurse is known as:
   a. Intuition *(circled)*
   b. Validation
   c. Reasoning
   d. Translating

5. Nurses are required to share data with their peers at each shift change. This shift-change communication must include which of the following elements? Select all that apply.

   _✓_ Accurate information

   _✓_ Information concerning the client's personality

   _____ The nurse's personal feelings about the client

   _✓_ Information regarding the level of the client's family support

   _____ The nurse's opinions about the client's family background

6. What is the purpose of the nursing assessment?

   The nursing assessment helps to find out the best course of action for nursing care. Identify possible nursing diagnosis. Focus on a specific problem. Determine immediate needs. Identify Risks for complications

7. What environmental considerations should be included in the physical assessment?

   ~~scribbled out~~, Occupation, where they live, Religious beliefs, Lighting for the Room.

8. When approaching the client for the first time to perform an assessment, the nurse should take what preliminary steps?

Prepare for the assessment, ~~bere~~ establish rapport with the client.

✱ Check the chart
✱ body substance isolation

9. Which of the following behaviors is most associated with the working phase of the client interview?
   a. Establishment of the purpose of the interaction
   b. Establishment of rapport
   c. Identification of the client's immediate concerns
   d. Making sure the client feels that his or her concerns have been understood

10. Gender and religious affiliation are types of biographical data.
    a. True
    b. False

11. When assessing a client's chief complaint, the nurse must investigate what factors?

Location of symptoms, quality, quantity, chronology, setting, aggravating + alleviating factors, + associated factors.

12. A concept referring to the positive and negative behaviors a person uses to interact with the environment and maintain health is known as *Functional health* patterns.

Exercise 2

 CD-ROM Activity

 45 minutes

- Sign in to work at Pacific View Regional Hospital on the Skilled Nursing Floor for Period of Care 2. (*Note:* If you are already in the virtual hospital from a previous exercise, click on **Leave the Floor** and then **Restart the Program** to get to the sign-in window.)
- From the Patient List, select William Jefferson (Room 501).
- Click on **Get Report** and read the report.
- Click on **Go to Nurses' Station**.
- Click on **Chart** and then on **501**.
- Click on and review the **History and Physical** tab.

1. Match each of the following assessment techniques with its correct definition.

Technique	Definition
_d_ Inspection	a. The use of the fingertips to tap the body's surface and produce vibration and sound
_b_ Palpation	b. The use of the hands and sense of touch to gather information
_c_ Auscultation	c. The process of listening to sounds produced by the body
_a_ Percussion	d. A visual observation of the client's body, responses to questioning, and nonverbal behaviors

2. If a focused assessment were to be performed on William Jefferson, what systems would be targeted? (*Hint:* Refer to the History and Physical.)

   Cardiovascular, endocrine, central nervous system, genitourinary, blood

- Click on **Return to Nurses' Station**.
- Click on **501** at the bottom of the screen.
- Click on **Patient Care**.
- Click on **Head & Neck** and review the assessment data in each area.

3. Which manner of data collection is being used by the nurse to assess William Jefferson?

   Palpation, inspection. Head to toe

4. What tools will be needed to complete an assessment of William Jefferson?

No tools are necessary for the assessment the nurse did, but they could have used an otoscope, ophthalmoscope, tuning fork, + tounge blade. Also a snellen eye chart Blood glucose meter

5. When William Jefferson's skin assessment is performed, which of the following factors is true? Select all that apply.

✓ In dark-skinned persons, the lips, palms, and nail beds are commonly light-toned.

_____ Light-colored soles and palms are indicative of an underlying disorder.

✓ Peripheral cyanosis is best observed in the skin of the arms and legs.

✓ Cyanosis can be seen as grayish tones in darker-skinned individuals.

_____ Darkened areas over the sacrum should be reported for further evaluation of a coagulation disorder.

6. The presence of skin lesions must be documented using correct terminology. Match each of the following terms with the appropriate description.

Lesion type		Description
b	Rash	a. A thin, linear crack in the epidermis
d	Excoriation	b. A skin eruption characterized by macules, papules, vesicles, or erythema
a	Fissure	c. An open lesion extending deeper than the dermis
c	Ulcer	d. Removal of surface skin by scraping or rubbing

7. List any abnormal findings in the nurse's assessment of William Jefferson's head and neck.

diabetic Rentinopathy, mild hearing deficit in left ear, Mild deficit of ROM of neck, hair coarse + dry, oriented to time + person only, impaired ST memory, confusion + agitation w/ unfamiliar ppl + situations, ↑ confusion since last assessment, difficulty w/ word finding, + impaired congnitive + perceptual ability.

8. What clues can be obtained from examination of the mouth and teeth?

hygiene ; illness, age

9. When pupils are equal and reactive to light, what acronym is used?

PERRLA

10. What were the pupillary findings for William Jefferson?

equal + Reactive

→ • Click on **Chest** and review the assessment data in each area.

11. The best means to access the lower lobes of the lungs is *posterior* _____.

12. List any abnormal findings in the nursing assessment of William Jefferson's chest.

apical HR slightly irregular

13. Match each of the following adventitious lung sounds with its description.

Lung Sound	Description
b Crackles	*a.* Sounds produced by a narrowing in the airway passages
a Wheezes	*b.* Bubbling sounds that may be evidenced on inspection
c Pleural friction rubs	*c.* Sounds produced by inflammation in the pleural sac; may have a rubbing, grating, or friction sound

→ • Click on **Back & Spine** and review the assessment data in each area.

14. List any abnormal findings in the nurse's assessment of William Jefferson's back and spine.

None

➡ • Click on **Upper Extremities** and review the assessment data in each area.

15. Identify any unusual findings in the assessment of the upper extremities.

any scaly area on elbows, mild deficit of ROM in shoulders (radial pulse 2+ bilatterally).

[margin: Normal - weak strong, Normal 4-0, weak, strong]

16. During the assessment of the abdomen, the client's knees should be ~~straight~~ ~~out~~.   Slightly flexed

17. Which of the following is the optimal positioning of a client during an abdominal assessment?
    (a.) Supine
    b. Prone
    c. Trendelenburg — head↓

18. As you prepare to perform the assessment of William Jefferson's abdomen, review the sequencing of steps required. Put each of the actions below in order of priority.

	Action	Order in sequence
b	Auscultate for bowel sounds in each of the four quadrants.	a. First
c	Palpate for masses or other abnormalities.	b. Second
a	Visually inspect the abdomen for size, symmetry, and general appearance.	c. Third

19. At least __5__ minutes of assessment must be allowed before deciding that bowel sounds are absent.

➡ • Click on **Abdomen** and review the assessment data in each area.

20. What were the findings regarding William Jefferson's bowel sounds?

Sound ausculated in all 4 quadrants

BS4Q

→ • Click on **Lower Extremities** and review the assessment data in each area.

21. List any findings of interest in the assessment of William Jefferson's lower extremities.

Slightly mottled color of feet & toes, easily fatigued, favors left leg, ~~both sides~~ strength mildly impaired, mildly impair ROM in both hips, capillary refill sluggish, pedal pulses 1+ bilaterally, impaired sensation in both feet, & numbness & tingling on bottoms of both feet

22. How is the capillary refill test performed?

By pressing on fingers, toes, or another extremity & seeing how long it takes for the skin to turn back to regular color

23. What were the findings in regard to William Jefferson's capillary refill? What are potential causes of this finding?

He has impaired capillary refill & it is probably cause by poor peripheral circulation caused by diabetes

→ • Click on **Patient Care** and then on **Nurse-Client Interactions**.
 • Select and view the video titled **1120: The Agitated Patient**. (*Note:* Check the virtual clock to see whether enough time has elapsed. You can use the fast-forward feature to advance the time by 2-minute intervals if the video is not yet available. Then click again on **Patient Care** and **Nurse-Client Interactions** to refresh the screen.)

24. How would you characterize William Jefferson's behavior In the video? What unique challenges will this behavior have for the nursing assessment?

He does not seem to be listening to the nurse or he is not comprehending it. The unique challenges the nurse will have during assessment may be having the client sit quietly. She may also may not be able to get close the client to palpate. She may not be able to get the client to follow directions as needed.

Assessment of Vital Signs

Reading Assignment: Assessing Vital Signs (Chapter 7)

Client: Kathryn Doyle, Skilled Nursing Floor, Room 503

Objectives:

1. Identify the rationale for the assessment of vital signs.
2. Interpret deviations from the normal ranges of each vital sign.
3. Describe the normal physiological features of each vital sign.
4. List factors that influence temperature, pulse, respirations, oxygen saturation, and blood pressure.

Exercise 1

Clinical Preparation: Writing Activity

30 minutes

1. Identify at least four situations in which vital sign assessment will benefit nursing care delivery. (*Hint:* See page 114 in your textbook.)

   - after surgery
   - to check effectiveness of interventions
   - routine monitoring
   - to establish a baseline

2. When interpreting vital signs, the readings cannot be considered in a vacuum. The vital signs must be reviewed for trends. What factors should be considered when making inferences about vital signs?

   Environmental factors, normal Ranges for the age group, baselines for the client, & clients complete history & condition.

3. ___*basal metabolic*___ rate represents the energy needed to maintain essential body functions expressed as calories per hour per square meter of body surface.

4. Normal body temperature ranges from ___*96.8*___ to ___*99.4*___ degrees Fahrenheit.

5. A woman has a slightly lower body temperature than a man.
   a. True
   b. False *(circled)*

6. Which of the following is correct regarding taking rectal temperature of an adult client?
   a. Position the client on the right side, not the left side, for better access to the client's anus.
   b. Left-side positioning is preferred for rectal temperature taking. *(circled)*
   c. Hold the thermometer in place for 4 to 6 minutes.
   d. Insert the thermometer about 1 inch into the rectum.

7. If a client has an elevated temperature, which of the following terms may be used to describe the client's condition? Select all that apply.

   _____ Afebrile

   _____ Hyposphresic

   _____ Febrile

   __✓__ Hyperthermic

   __✓__ Pyretic

8. A heart rate less than 60 beats per minute is known as ___*bradycardia*___.

9. List several factors that may influence heart rate.

   ANS, medications, low blood pressure, dehydration, fever, pain

10. The preferred location for pulse assessment in the child or infant younger than 2 years is

    brachial .

11. Match each of the following breathing patterns with its correct description.

Pattern		Description
_d._	Eupnea	a. Rate and depth are increased, associated with diabetic ketoacidosis
_b._	Bradypnea	b. Regular rhythm of less than 12 breaths per minute in an adult
_f._	Tachypnea	c. Alternating periods of apnea, hypoventilation, and hyperventilation, associated with a head injury or heart failure
_e._	Apnea	
_a._	Kussmaul	d. Rate between 12 and 20 breaths per minute with regular rhythm and moderate depth
_c._	Cheyne-Stokes	e. Absence or respirations leading to respiratory arrest and death
		f. Regular rhythm of more than 20 breaths per minute of an adult

12. Normal oxygen saturation is between _95_ % and _100_ %.

13. When taking the blood pressure, the bell of the stethoscope should be placed over the radial artery.
    a. True
    (b.) False

14. Normal blood pressure is between __110__ and __130__ mm Hg systolic and _60_ and _80_ mm Hg diastolic.

15. Considering the potential causes of errors in blood pressure readings, which of the following may be associated with false low readings? Select all that apply.

    _✓_ Cuff size too wide

    ____ Cuff size too narrow

    _✓_ Cuff wrapped too loosely

    _✓_ Arm above heart level

    _✓_ Failure to wait at least 30 to 60 seconds between blood pressure readings

    _✓_ Manometer below eye level

Exercise 2

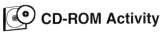 **CD-ROM Activity**

 45 minutes

- Sign in to work at Pacific View Regional Hospital on the Skilled Nursing Floor for Period of Care 1. (*Note:* If you are already in the virtual hospital from a previous exercise, click on **Leave the Floor** and then **Restart the Program** to get to the sign-in window.)
- From the Patient List, select Kathryn Doyle (Room 503).
- Click on **Get Report** and read the report.
- Click on **Go to Nurses' Station** then on **503** at the bottom of the screen.
- Click on **Take Vital Signs**.

1. What are Kathryn Doyle's vital signs?

Temperature: 102°F

Blood pressure: 115/75

Heart rate: 101

Respirations: 21

2. Discuss any abnormal findings in the above vital signs.

high temp, just above normal HR + Resp.

3. Based on your knowledge of Kathryn Doyle's health history, to what might her elevated temperature be attributed?

May be due to infection b/c of hip Replacement, or may be caused by ↓ in fluid.

4. What interventions may be used to treat Kathryn Doyle's temperature elevation?

Take off blankets open doors, drink fluids

5. The elevation in Kathryn Doyle's temperature will be accompanied by a decreased heart rate.
   a. True
   b. False *(circled)*

6. If a nursing assistant is available to assist in taking Kathryn Doyle's vital signs, which of the following statements is *most* correct?
   a. The nursing assistant may be delegated the responsibility of taking the vital signs.
   b. Since there is an abnormality in Kathryn Doyle's vital signs, the nursing assistant should not be delegated to work with this particular client.
   c. The nursing assistant may take the vital signs, but charting the findings is the responsibility of the nurse.
   d. Although the nursing assistant may be delegated the responsibility of taking the vital signs, the nurse is still responsible for monitoring the results. *(circled)*

→ • Click on **Patient Care** and then on **Nurse-Client Interactions**.
   • Select and view the video titled **0730: Assessment—Biopsychosocial**. (*Note:* Check the virtual clock to see whether enough time has elapsed. You can use the fast-forward feature to advance the time by 2-minute intervals if the video is not yet available. Then click again on **Patient Care** and **Nurse-Client Interactions** to refresh the screen.)

7. In the video, what actions and/or statements by Kathryn Doyle support the elevated temperature finding?

   "Awfully tired"
   "As weak as newborn kitten"
   "don't feel right"
   "don't feel like myself"

8. Discuss the impact that Kathryn Doyle's elevated temperature will have on the frequency of her assessments.

   Because she is @ risk for complications caused by elevated temp, she will be checked more often.

9. Which of the following actions should the nurse take prior to reporting the elevation in Kathryn Doyle's temperature? Select all that apply.

   ✓ Recheck the temperature to ensure proper functioning of equipment.

   _____ Administer acetaminophen.

   ✓ Check physician's orders to determine whether call orders have been left.

_____ Ask a nursing assistant to recheck the temperature.

✓ Ask the client whether she had eaten just before her temperature was taken.

_____ Give the client a tepid sponge bath.

✓ Administer ordered antibiotics.

➡ • Click on **Chart** and then on **503**.
   • Click on the **Physician's Orders** tab and review the orders.

10. What orders has the physician left regarding Kathryn Doyle's temperature?

Acetaminophen every 4 hrs for mild fever

11. Prior to administering acetaminophen, what actions should the nurse take?

Check equipment, make sure the patient did not drink, eat, or smoke before temp was assessed, check temp again if needed

12. Which of Kathryn Doyle's prescribed medications may have had an impact on her current temperature? Select all that apply.

_____ Ferrous sulfate

✓ Calcium citrate

✗ Ibuprofen

_____ Docusate sodium

✗ Oxycodone

✗ Acetaminophen

13. How will acetaminophen reduce Kathryn Doyle's temperature?

B/c it is an antipyretic

14. How soon should Kathryn Doyle's temperature be retaken once she is given acetaminophen? Why?

> 30-60 minutes after so the medication has time to work

15. Identify two nursing diagnoses that would be applicable to Kathryn Doyle's health status and her abnormal vital signs?

> 1) Elevated Respirations & heart Rate
> 2) Low-grade fever

Development of the Nursing Care Plan

Reading Assignment: Planning, Intervening, and Evaluation (Chapter 10)

Client: William Jefferson, Skilled Nursing Floor, Room 501

Objectives:

1. Describe the types of planning for individual clients.
2. Identify the process of planning expected outcomes and interventions.
3. Discuss the categories and types of interventions to individualize care for each client.
4. Describe the development of a nursing care plan.

Exercise 1

Clinical Preparation: Writing Activity

 15 minutes

1. Match each of the following aspects of the nursing process with its appropriate description.

Nursing Process Step	Description
_c_ Assess	a. Set goals and desired outcomes
_a_ Plan and identify outcomes	b. Identify the client's problems
_e_ Intervention	c. Gather information about the client's condition
_d_ Evaluation	d. Determine whether goals are met and outcomes have been achieved
_b_ Diagnosis	e. Perform the nursing actions identified in planning

2. How do medical and nursing diagnoses differ?

   Medical dx = etiologies + disease processes

   Nursing dx = the illnesses effects on the person

3. When the nurse collects data about the client, what are sources of information other than the client?

   family/friends, medical records, other Health care personnel

4. Maslow's hierarchy is used to establish priorities. Identify the level of each stage listed below.

	Stage of Maslow's Hierarchy	**Level**
3	Love and belonging	a. Level 1
1	Basic physiological needs	a. Level 2
5	Self-actualization	a. Level 3
2	Safety and security	a. Level 4
4	Self esteem	a. Level 5

5. *Consultation* ~~Collaboration~~ is the act of two or more health care professionals, one of whom is an expert or specialist, solicited to offer an opinion for the purpose of making decisions.

6. Two or more health care professionals performing together to achieve a common goal is known as *Collaboration* .

7. Indicate whether each of the following statements is true or false.

   a. *F* Case management plans are implemented to reduce nursing workload and improve nursing job satisfaction.

   b. *T* A clinical pathway can provide a means to coordinate care and reduce costs.

Standardized Care plans)

Case Management plans

8. If a care plan has been developed by a graduate nurse, which of the following client outcomes is appropriate?
   a. The nurse will evaluate the temperature every 4 hours.
   b. The physician will prescribe antibiotics as indicated.
   c. The client will exhibit a reduction in temperature within 24 hours.
   d. The family will understand the treatment plan.

Exercise 2

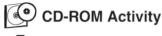 **CD-ROM Activity**

 45 minutes

• Sign in to work at Pacific View Regional Hospital on the Skilled Nursing Floor for Period of Care 3. (*Note:* If you are already in the virtual program from a previous exercise, click on **Leave the Floor** and then **Restart the Program** to get to the sign-in window.)
• From the Patient List, select William Jefferson (Room 501).
• Click on **Get Report** and read the report.
• Click on **Go to Nurses' Station**.
• Click on **Chart** and then on **501**.
• Click on and review the **Nursing Admission** tab.

1. Who appears to be the primary provider of information in the nursing admission assessment of William Jefferson?

   His wife ~~name~~ ←signed power of attorney

2. Identify the primary concerns reported by the client.

   If he is getting worse + when is he going home

3. Which of the following have been identified as medical diagnoses for William Jefferson? Select all that apply.

   __✓__ Alzheimer's disease

   _____ Stress incontinence

   __✓__ Urinary tract infection

   __✓__ Hypertension

_____ ✓ Potential for anxiety

~~_____~~ Osteoporosis

_____ ✓ Type 2 diabetes mellitus

_____ Diabetes insipidus

_____ ✓ Resolving sepsis

_____ ✓ Osteoarthritis

➤ • Click on and review the **History and Physical** tab.

4. Based on information collected in the Nursing Admission and the History and Physical, identify several areas of concern for William Jefferson.

Management of diabetes + hypertension. Inability to do some activities @ home. Functional decline from ADL+ delirium.

5. Below is a list of nursing diagnoses based on functional health patterns. Select all diagnoses that are applicable to the needs of William Jefferson.

_____ Health-seeking behaviors

_____ Risk for infection

_____ ✓ Risk for injury

_____ Adult failure to thrive

_____ ✓ Anxiety

_____ ✓ Acute confusion

_____ ✓ Deficient knowledge

6. Develop a client outcome related to William Jefferson's potential for injury.

Client + family will list ways to prevent injuries @ home by discharge. The client will remain free from injury

7. Develop a client outcome related to William Jefferson's diabetes mellitus.

Client will maintain BG levels w/in normal limits

The client will demonstrate how to give an insulin shot by discharge.

or

Clients blood sugar will decrease to 200 by 3 day

→ • Click on the **Physician's Orders** tab and review the orders for Tuesday at 1230.

8. How do nursing interventions and physician-prescribed interventions differ?

Physicians orders ~~are mainly~~ ~~what was going on~~ are more about medical interventions while nurses orders may include the clients abilities, feelings, + working w/ client

9. Which of the orders listed below are nursing interventions? Select all that apply.

✓ Temperature, pulse, respirations daily only

▓ Fingerstick capillary glucose at bedtime tonight

___ Fasting blood glucose Wednesday morning

✓ Continue blood pressure check every 8 hours

→ • Click on the **Consultations** tab and review the data.

10. Why are multiple disciplines utilized to provide care to William Jefferson?

Physical / Occupational therapy

11. What consultations have been made so far in William Jefferson's care?

Mon + Tues, ROM + Resistance/ Strength training

12. Based on the data presented concerning William Jefferson's physical condition and psychosocial needs, which of the following consultations would be helpful to him and to his family? Select all that apply.

✓ Support groups

✓ Respite care resources *= "Vacation"*

_____ Hospice services

_____ Respiratory therapy

~~✗~~ Cardiovascular rehabilitation

✓ Dietary services

Documenting Care

 Reading Assignment: Documenting Care (Chapter 11)

Client: Jacquline Catanazaro, Medical-Surgical Floor, Room 402

Objectives:

1. Understand the purposes of documentation.
2. Identify the methods of implementation of the principles of documentation.
3. Identify content pertinent to various types of nursing entries, special populations, and facilities.
4. Differentiate among documentation formats and the usefulness of various types of flow sheets.
5. Apply the principles of documentation to electronic documentation systems.

Exercise 1

 CD-ROM Activity

45 minutes

1. List the five purposes of documentation.

   a. Communication

   b. quality assurance

   c. legal accountability

   d. Reimbursement

   e. Research

2. While working on the nursing unit, a nurse who has already gone home calls back to the floor and reports that she has forgotten to note the client's activity during her shift. Which of the following actions by the nurse currently on the unit is most appropriate?
   a. Agree to note the client's activities and sign the other nurse's signature
   b. Contact the nursing supervisor
   c. Advise the nurse you will pass on her concerns but you will not document the information in her absence
   d. Refuse to become involved

3. While documenting a client's treatment, the nurse realizes he has made an error in the information recorded. Which of the following actions by the nurse is most appropriate?
   a. Erase the information that was recorded in error.
   b. Obtain a new flow sheet and start the page over.
   c. Use a permanent marker and completely cover the information recorded in error.
   d. Call the nursing supervisor.
   e. Neatly draw a single line through the error and record the correct information.

4. Match each of the following root words, prefixes, and suffixes used in documentation with its correct meaning.

Word Part		Meaning
f	Adeno	a. Cell
a	Cyto	b. Blood
k	Derma	c. Difficult, painful
i	Osteo	d. Many, multiple
g	Patho	e. Deficiency; lack of
j	Hemi-	f. Gland
l	Uni-	g. Disease
c	Dys-	h. Discharge
d	Poly-	i. Bone
m	-Cele	j. Half
b	-Emia	k. Skin
e	-Penia	l. One
h	-Rhea	m. Swelling, protrusion

5. When charting information, the nurse realizes an entry from the previous shift has not been included. The nurse who omitted the information has left the facility and will not be available until the next day. Which action is most appropriate to manage this situation?
   a. The nurse who did not document in a timely manner can write the information in the margins around the time of events.
   b. The nurse who is currently documenting should leave a few lines blank for the other nurse to document at a later date.
   c. The nurse should continue to document findings and actions and the late entries can be entered as addendums.
   d. Late information cannot be listed in the permanent file after 24 hours.

6. An ___admit___ or ___admission___ note is the nurse's first documentation for a new client who has just entered the facility.

7. Interval or ___Progress___ notes are interdisciplinary notes entered at various times during a shift.

8. A transfer note is used when one nurse goes off duty and transfers the client's care to another nurse.   _When transferring to another_
   a. True   _facility or to another part of hospital_
   b. False

Change of shift notes are when a nurse is going off shift

9. The nurse is admitting a client to the unit from the physician's office. The nurse notes that the client is wearing several pieces of expensive jewelry. What are the responsibilities of the nurse in this matter?

   The nurse must give a detailed description of the items on the outside of the envelop in which they will be placed. An entry note must also be made that the items were received + where they have been sent. May require signatures of 2 HC professionals w/ Copy placed in chart   Must also doc. name of + Relationship of person if items are sent home w/ someone else.

10. In APIE (PIE) charting, what does the acronym stand for?

    A: Assessment
    P: ~~Planning~~ Problem ID   *Planning*
    I: implementation
    E: evaluation

11. When SOAP charting is used in a facility, the nurse should be aware of the acronym's meaning. Identify the parts of SOAP charting.

    S: subjective data

    O: objective data

    A: Assessment

    P: Plan

12. It is the choice of the nurse whether to use military time or AM/PM.
    a. True
    b. False   Military

13. What is the role of nursing informatics?

    ensuring nursing's data & knowledge are structured in such a way that they can be understood & used by other members of the HCT.

14. What is an electronic health record (EHR)?

    Comprehensive Record of a clients Cure across different facilities and/or admissions

15. What is HIPAA, and how does it affect documentation?

    HIPAA = Health Insurance Portability & Accountability Act.

    places
    Affect doc. by limiting transfer of info. & protecting patients rights
    Added protection. HC providers have passwords

Exercise 2

 CD-ROM Activity

30 minutes

- Sign in to work at Pacific View Regional Hospital on the Medical-Surgical Floor for Period of Care 2. (*Note:* If you are already in the virtual hospital from a previous exercise, click on **Leave the Floor** and then **Restart the Program** to get to the sign-in window.)
- From the Patient List, select Jacquline Catanazaro (Room 402).
- Click on **Get Report** and read the report.
- Click on **Go to Nurses' Station** and then on **402** at the bottom of the screen.
- Read the **Initial Observations**.
- Click on **Take Vital Signs**.

1. What type of documentation form would be used to record the vital signs taken for Jacquline Catanazaro?

   Flow sheet, doc. Routine assessment data.
   ⋆ Graphic Sheet ⋆

2. The Initial Observation report at 1115 is an example of what type of documentation?

   Narrative

3. Jacquline Catanazaro has an IV. What information concerning the IV will need to be included in documentation relating to it?

   The fluid being admin., Rate of flow, correct placement, ensure they are secured. Should check site for tenderness, Redness, edema, & warmth. IV should be assessed @ least every 2 hr. IV site should be documented.

→ - Click on **Patient Care** and then on **Nurse-Client Interactions**.
- Select and view the video titled **1115: Assessment—Readiness to Learn**. (*Note:* Check the virtual clock to see whether enough time has elapsed. You can use the fast-forward feature to advance the time by 2-minute intervals if the video is not yet available. Then click again on **Patient Care** and **Nurse-Client Interactions** to refresh the screen.)

4. Jacquline Catanazaro has voiced a desire to wait to have teaching concerning her care. What should be recorded in the progress notes concerning this interaction?

1115 Went in for teaching of MDI. Wished to have sister present. ~~Wait until sister arrives.~~ Voiced concern w/ remembering info. Will wait until sister arrives.

5. When documenting Jacquline Catanazaro's response during the interaction, which of the following statements should be included in the progress notes? Select all that apply.

- ~~✓~~ The client refused the teaching.
- ___ Teaching was completed.
- ✓ Attempted to initiate MDI education.
- ___ The client is not receptive to receiving MDI education.
- ✓ The client asks to have her sister present to participate in the teaching session.

6. When the MDI education is performed, what factors should the nurse record?

- ✓ Completion of teaching
- ~~✓~~ Length of time required to perform teaching
- ✓ Client's level of understanding of information provided
- ✓ Time the teaching was performed
- ___ Expiration date for the MDI used in the session
- ✓ Family members include in the teaching session

→ • Click **Physical Assessment** and perform a head-to-toe assessment.

7. Which of the body systems reviewed will require documentation if a focus charting approach is being used?

Respiratory - Mild Tachypnea, crackles in RLL, productive cough, mild hyperresonance

MS
Mental

8. Which of the following statements about charting by exception are correct? Select all that apply.

___✓___ Reduces duplication

_____ Facilitates identification of omissions in care

___✓___ Limits amount of details

_____ Promotes following the nursing process

___✓___ Well-suited to the electronic medical record

9. Which of the following statements concerning Jacquline Catanazaro's assessment should be included in the permanent medical record? Select all that apply.

_____ 1120 a.m.—Respiratory system ok.

___✓___ 1120—Respiratory efforts normal.

_____ AM assessment—Jackie is coughing up white spit.

___✓___ 1120—Productive cough with frothy white sputum.

_____ 11:20 a.m.—Good respiratory efforts noted.

10. Using the SOAP format, document Jacquline Catanazaro's respiratory status assessment.

S:

O: Crackling in RLL, productive white sputum (More info.)

A: client has impaired No change

P: Admin O₂, Continue Meds as ordered

11. What are the disadvantages of using the SOAP format for charting?

Lack of flexibility

12. If charting by exception were employed to document findings on Jacquline Catanazaro's abdomen, a notation would be required.
a. True
b. False ← correct

- Click on **Patient Care** and then on **Nurse-Client Interactions**.
- Select and view the video titled **1140: Compliance—Medications**. (*Note:* Check the virtual clock to see whether enough time has elapsed. You can use the fast-forward feature to advance the time by 2-minute intervals if the video is not yet available. Then click again on **Patient Care** and **Nurse-Client Interactions** to refresh the screen.)

13. Prepare a narrative notation for the medical record detailing the events that took place during the interaction.

> 1140: Teaching w/ client. Sister present. *[illegible]* patient about *[illegible]* medication. Became frustrated when trying to administer on own. Upset about weight gain from previous medication. *[illegible]* Willing to change diet *[illegible]* to lose weight. Teaching not complete

- Click on **EPR** and then on **Login**.
- Select **402** as the patient and **Vital Signs** as the category.
- Review the notations for Wednesday.

14. The EPR has a notation indicating the Nurse's Notes should be reviewed concerning characteristics of pain being experienced by Jacquline Catanazaro. What documentation relating to this notation is present in the nurse's notes?

> Wed 0705
> gave pain meds
> None

LESSON **7**

The Nurse-Client Relationship

 Reading Assignment: The Nurse-Client Relationship (Chapter 12)

Client: William Jefferson, Skilled Nursing Floor, Room 501

Objectives:

1. Describe the nature of a therapeutic relationship.
2. Identify nursing attitudes that promote therapeutic communication.
3. Describe phases of the nurse-client relationship.
4. Discuss effective therapeutic communication techniques.
5. Discuss nontherapeutic communication techniques.

Exercise 1

 CD-ROM Activity

30 minutes

1. List the roles of the nurse in a therapeutic relationship with a client. (*Hint:* Refer to the roles outlined by Hildegard Peplau.)

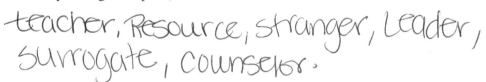

teacher, Resource, stranger, Leader, surrogate, counselor.

2. Match each of the following types of feedback with its appropriate description.

Feedback	Description
_b_ Internal	a. Affirms efforts to communicate
_d_ External	b. A mechanism of self-perception
_a_ Positive	c. Responses by the client that indicate the messages sent were poorly transmitted or not well received
_c_ Negative	d. Received from another or others in the form of visual, auditory, or kinesthetic information

3. Identify the elements of nonverbal communication.

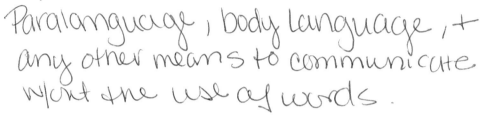

Paralanguage, body language, + any other means to communicate w/out the use of words.

4. _paralanguage_ refers to nonverbal components of spoken language.

5. The nurse is providing education to a client regarding the use of medications after discharge. Which of the following interpersonal space zones should be observed?
   a. Public space
   b. Social space
   c. Intimate space
   d. Personal space

6. Indicate whether each of the following statements is true or false.

   a. __T__ The nurse who experiences a sense of sadness with the client who has suffered a miscarriage is demonstrating empathy.

   b. __F__ The terms empathy and sympathy are interchangable.

7. A nurse who has a history of cervical cancer is caring for a client who has just found out she has cervical cancer in situ. Which of the following terms best describes the nurse's ability to share her own experiences with the client?
   a. Sympathy
   b. Relatedness
   c. Empathy
   d. Caring

8. A nurse prepares to discharge a client after a lengthy hospitalization. At the time of discharge, the client warmly clasps the nurse in a hearty handshake and hug. The nurse smiles and pats the client on the back. What behavior is being demonstrated by the nurse?
   a. Openness
   b. Professional closeness
   c. Caring
   d. Genuineness *(circled)*

9. ___Therapeutic Rapport___ is a special bond between a nurse and a client who have established a sense of trust and mutual understanding of the expectations in their relationship.

10. While completing the admission assessment, the client briefly mentions having been ill with similar symptoms several years ago. What communication technique should be employed by the nurse in this situation?
    a. Exploring *(circled)*
    b. Focusing
    c. Provide silence
    d. Reflection

11. Match each of the following nontherapeutic communication techniques with its appropriate description.

    Technique

    _c_ Interpreting

    _d_ Disagreeing

    _e_ Disapproving

    _a_ Parroting

    _b_ False reassurance

    Description

    a. Mechanically repeating the client's words without evaluating what has been said

    b. Implication that there is no cause for worry or concern

    c. An attempt to advise the client of the meaning of the client's experience

    d. Implication that the client is wrong

    e. A negate value judgment concerning the client's behavior or thoughts

12. When does the process of client education begin?
    (scribbled out text) Working Phase

13. At the time the client is admitted to the acute care facility, what information should be provided regarding the environment? ?

Lighting, space

Exercise 2

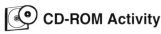 **CD-ROM Activity**

 45 minutes

- Sign in to work at Pacific View Regional Hospital on the Skilled Nursing Floor for Period of Care 1. (*Note:* if you are already in the virtual hospital from a previous exercise, click on **Leave the Floor** and then **Restart the Program** to get to the sign-in window.)
- From the Patient List, select William Jefferson (Room 501).
- Click on **Get Report** and read the report.
- Click on **Go to Nurses' Station** and then on **501**.
- Read the **Initial Observations**.

1. What psychosocial issues could affect the nurse's interaction with William Jefferson? How might these behaviors affect the interaction?

Mr. Jefferson is anxious & confused. & looking for his wife & dog. The nurse may need to use techniques for calming the client. The nurse may also need to use the technique of presenting reality. The nurse will need to use techniques to communicate w/ client.

2. What physiological and environmental issues being experienced by William Jefferson may affect the nurse-client interaction?

B/c he is unaware of where he is & why he may need reminding in a caring way.

3. Which of the following interventions will assist the nurse in establishing a positive rapport when communicating with William Jefferson? Select all that apply.

_____ Assist the client to the dining room to promote feelings of socialization.

✓ Face him during the interaction.

_____ Avoid analgesic administration to reduce drowsiness during the interaction.

✓ Provide adequate lighting during the exchange.

_____ Use touch as culturally appropriate.

4. When the nurse is caring for William Jefferson, which of the following variables will have the most influence on communication?
   a. His age and race
   b. His culture and social position
   c. The scheduled agenda for the day
   d. The race of the care provider
   (e) His disorientation and confusion

➡ • Click on **Patient Care** and then on **Nurse-Client Interactions**.
   • Select and view the video titled **0730: Intervention—Patient Safety**. (*Note:* Check the virtual clock to see whether enough time has elapsed. You can use the fast-forward feature to advance the time by 2-minute intervals if the video is not yet available. Then click again on **Patient Care** and **Nurse-Client Interactions** to refresh the screen.)

5. Review and critique the nurse's interaction with William Jefferson. What behaviors does the nurse exhibit in attempting to establish a rapport with him?

She helps the client to move. She also communicates w/ him about his wife. She seems a little frustrated. Her tone did not sound very caring. She was more worried about safety; did not ask about wife or his feelings

6. Which of the following is the primary concern for the nurse during the interaction?

_____✓_____ The safety of the client

_____ The client's disorientation

_____ Locating the client's family members

_____ The client's ability to tolerate ambulation

⟶ • Click on **Patient Care** and then on **Nurse-Client Interactions**.
• Select and view the video titled **0740: The Confused Patient**. (*Note:* Check the virtual clock to see whether enough time has elapsed. You can use the fast-forward feature to advance the time by 2-minute intervals if the video is not yet available. Then click again on **Patient Care** and **Nurse-Client Interactions** to refresh the screen.)

7. During the nurse-client interaction, the nurse is working within the client's space. Which of the following space zones is being used by the nurse?
a. Intimate
b. Personal
c. Social
d. Public

8. During the interaction, what communication techniques are used by the nurse?

Presenting Reality, offering self

9. The nurse's initial attempts to touch William Jefferson are rebuffed. Are her repeated attempts appropriate?

No

⟶ • Click on **Patient Care** and then on **Nurse-Client Interactions**.
• Select and view the video titled **0745: Intervention—Redirection**. (*Note:* Check the virtual clock to see whether enough time has elapsed. You can use the fast-forward feature to advance the time by 2-minute intervals if the video is not yet available. Then click again on **Patient Care** and **Nurse-Client Interactions** to refresh the screen.)

10. What is the primary underlying purpose of the communication technique being demonstrated by the nurse during the interaction?
   a. Distraction
   b. Assessment of cognition
   c. Assessment of client's personal interests
   d. Evaluation of client's needs

11. Review William Jefferson's appearance and behaviors during the interaction with the nurse. Describe them for each of the elements listed below. (*Hint:* You can replay the video if needed.)

Personal appearance: *Looks well groomed as far as hygiene. Shirt untucked but looks decent*

Facial expression: *happy about the fishing mag. upset about not knowing where wife & dog are.*

Eye contact: *Good eye contact.*

Exercise 3

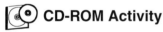 **CD-ROM Activity**

 30 minutes

- Sign in to work at Pacific View Regional Hospital in the Skilled Nursing Floor for Period of Care 2. (*Note:* If you are already in the virtual hospital from a previous exercise, click on **Leave the Floor** and then **Restart the Program** to get to the sign-in window.)
- From the Patient List, select William Jefferson (Room 501).
- Click on **Get Report** and read the report.

1. What cognitive changes took place in William Jefferson during the last shift?

Became confused w/ anxiety. Became aggressive & combative when comfort offered. No knowledge of place & situation. Poor participation.

2. What behavioral manifestations are occurring as a result of these changes?

Combative, aggressive, no participation in activities

➤ • Click on **Go to Nurses' Station** and then on **501**.
  • Review the **Initial Observations**.
  • Click on **Patient Care** and then on **Nurse-Client Interactions**.
  • Select and view the video titled **1115: Team Communication**. (*Note:* Check the virtual clock to see whether enough time has elapsed. You can use the fast-forward feature to advance the time by 2-minute intervals if the video is not yet available. Then click again on **Patient Care** and **Nurse-Client Interactions** to refresh the screen.)

3. What is the primary nursing intervention discussed in the team conference that will be implemented by the nurse?

To find out what else could be causing the behavior besides an unfamiliar environment.

4. Provide a rationale for the above planned intervention.

Maybe there is something else bothering him or maybe he is having serious cognitive abilities.

5. After the nurse assesses for potential causes of William Jefferson's increasing levels of agitation, which of the following activities can be used to assess for potential sources of his concerns? Select all that apply.

____✓____ Schedule a conference with the client's family.

____✓____ Review the medications being administered to the client.

____✓____ Monitor the client's vital signs.

____✓____ Review the client's permanent medical record.

• Click on **Patient Care** and then on **Nurse-Client Interactions**.

• Select and view the video titled **1120: The Agitated Patient**. (*Note:* Check the virtual clock to see whether enough time has elapsed. You can use the fast-forward feature to advance the time by 2-minute intervals if the video is not yet available. Then click again on **Patient Care** and **Nurse-Client Interactions** to refresh the screen.)

6. The nurse is able to successfully reorient William Jefferson.
   a. True
   b. False

7. Identify the communication techniques used by the nurse.

   _____✓_____ Reorientation

   _____✓_____ Therapeutic touch

   _____ Sympathy

   _____ Hugging

   _____✓_____ Distraction

8. Which of the following factors associated with the client's room may affect communication?
   a. Color of the room
   b. Size of the room
   c. Physical layout of the room
   d. Lack of a roommate

LESSON **8**

Client Teaching

Reading Assignment: Client Teaching (Chapter 13)

Client: Clarence Hughes, Medical-Surgical Floor, Room 404

Objectives:

1. Explain the rationale for client teaching, including its purpose and benefits.
2. Describe the teaching and learning process, including domains of learning and principles of effective teaching.
3. Describe factors that affect client teaching.
4. Explore strategies for effectively implementing client teaching.
5. Discuss methods for evaluating teaching and learning.
6. Develop individualized nursing diagnoses related to the educational needs of clients.
7. Implement changes in the teaching plans for the client experiencing complications.

Exercise 1

 Clinical Preparation: Writing Activity

 30 minutes

1. A student nurse asks the nursing instructor why there is so much emphasis on client teaching. Which of the following should be included in the instructor's response to the student? Select all that apply.

   _____ Client teaching increases the overall costs of hospitalization.

   _____ Client teaching can reduce the reoccurrences of illness.

   _____ Client teaching promotes the client's ability to control his or her own care.

   _____ Client teaching can reduce the need for costly medical procedures.

2. The provision of client teaching is primarily the responsibility of the nursing team.
   a. True
   b. False

3. _____ is a set of planned activities preformed to influence knowledge, behavior or skill.

4. Match each of the following domains of learning with its correct definition.

Domain of Learning	**Definition**
_____ Cognitive	a. Manipulative and motor skills
_____ Affective	b. The ability to understand and use information presented
_____ Psychomotor	c. Feelings and values affiliated with information

5. The nurse is preparing to teach a 10-year-old child about caring for her arm cast. Which of the following means will be most effective?
   a. Role playing
   b. Providing a written list of instructions
   c. Using a model to demonstrate cast care
   d. Engaging the child in a discussion in which they are allowed to use problem-solving techniques

6. Identify the common age-related learning needs that may be present in a 14-year-old female. Select all that apply.

   _____ Nutrition and exercise

   _____ Stress management

   _____ Dental hygiene

   _____ Self-esteem

   _____ Safety

   _____ Substance abuse

7. Which of the following are principles associated with adult learning? Select all that apply.

_____ Motivated most by external sources

_____ Builds on previous knowledge

_____ Desire to use knowledge at a much later date

_____ Practical

_____ Purposeful

_____ Self-directed

8. The nurse is preparing to provide discharge teaching to a client who voices an inability to "take all of this in right now." What action should the nurse take first?
   a. Contact the physician.
   b. Agree to postpone the session for a brief period of time.
   c. Provide the client with written instructions to review after discharge.
   d. Advise the client to contact the hospital after discharge if questions/concerns arise.

9. Identify five types of barriers that can inhibit learning.

10. _____ _____ is the nursing diagnosis that applies when the client lacks knowledge of health management practices needed to achieve or maintain health.

Exercise 2

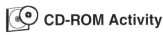 **CD-ROM Activity**

 45 minutes

- Sign in to work at Pacific View Regional Hospital on the Medical-Surgical Floor for Period of Care 1. (*Note:* If you are already in the virtual hospital from a previous exercise, click on **Leave the Floor** and then **Restart the Program** to get to the sign-in window.)
- From the Patient List, select Clarence Hughes (Room 404).

1. Match each of the following client activities to the correct domain of learning.

Client Activity	**Domain of Learning**
_____ Understanding the schedule for analgesics during the postoperative period	a. Cognitive
_____ Ability to use assistive devices correctly	b. Affective
_____ Knowledge of signs and symptoms to report after discharge	c. Psychomotor
_____ Understanding the need to rely on others for help after discharge	

- Click on **Get Report** and read the report.
- Click on **Go to Nurses' Station** and then on **404** at the bottom of the screen.
- Review the **Initial Observations**.
- Click on and review **Clinical Alerts**.
- Click on **Patient Care** and then on **Nurse-Client Interactions**.
- Select and view the videos titled **0730: Assessment—Perception of Care** and **0740: Empathy**. (*Note:* Check the virtual clock to see whether enough time has elapsed. You can use the fast-forward feature to advance the time by 2-minute intervals if the videos are not yet available. Then click again on **Patient Care** and **Nurse-Client Interactions** to refresh the screen.)

2. Identify the teaching needs for Clarence Hughes at this time. Select all that apply.

_____ Pain management

_____ Management of constipation

_____ Eating a balanced diet

_____ Prevention of osteoarthritis

3. Identify potential barriers to Clarence Hughes' readiness for discharge teaching.

- Click on **Chart** and then on **404**.
- Click on and review the **Physician's Notes** tab.

4. What is the physician's plan of care, according to the note on Wednesday 0700?

5. Identify family members and health care providers who need to be included in the plan of care.

6. In preparation for discharge, the nurse should rely on Clarence Hughes' level of education to determine the level of written materials to provide.
   a. True
   b. False

7. When assessing readiness to learn, the nurse should pose which of the following questions to Clarence Hughes to best assess his level of motivation?
   a. "Are you ready to go home?"
   b. "What has your physician told you about being discharged?"
   c. "What are your main concerns about the discharge?"
   d. "Will you have help at home?"

8. Listed below are possible causes of deficient knowledge. Which of the factors are currently applicable to Clarence Hughes?

   _____   Cognitive limitation

   _____   Information misinterpretation

   _____   Lack of interest in learning

   _____   Lack of readiness to learn

   _____   Lack of recall

   _____   Limited exposure to information

   _____   Limited practice of skill

   _____   Unfamiliarity with information resources

9. Select the correctly stated learning objective for Clarence Hughes.
   a. The nurse will provide education concerning the date of discharge.
   b. The client will understand the teaching provided.
   c. The client will verbalize correct use of analgesics prescribed after discharge.
   d. The nurse will identify the goals for the client's teaching session.

➜ • Click on and review the **Patient Education** tab.

10. After his pain is within tolerable limits, what teaching needs are present for Clarence Hughes?

➜ • Clarence Hughes' physician has ordered enoxaparin therapy to continue after discharge.
   • Click on **Return to Room 404**.
   • Click on the **Drug** icon to access the Drug Guide for information relating to this medication.

11. Identify the information that will need to be presented to Clarence Hughes concerning the enoxaparin. Select all that apply.

_____ Method of administration

_____ Adverse reactions that may occur

_____ Adverse reactions to report

_____ Other indications for medication usage

_____ Dosage range for the adult population

12. What is the best means to evaluate Clarence Hughes' level of understanding concerning home administration of enoxaparin?
    a. Return demonstration by the client
    b. Verbalization by client of his understanding of the medication's use
    c. Verbalization by family members that they understand the medication's use
    d. Willingness of client to sign the discharge teaching sheet

13. Match each of the following client responses to the correct component of the cognitive domain.

Response	Cognitive Domain Component
_____ "I understand why I need to use this CPM machine."	a. Acquisition
	b. Comprehension
_____ "I would rather have a pill instead of a suppository to help me have a bowel movement."	c. Application
	d. Analysis
_____ "The pain medication helped me to rest."	e. Synthesis
	f. Evaluation

Exercise 3

 CD-ROM Activity

 15 minutes

- Sign in to work at Pacific View Regional Hospital on the Medical-Surgical Floor for Period of Care 2. (*Note:* If you are already in the virtual hospital from a previous exercise, click on **Leave the Floor** and then **Restart the Program** to get to the sign-in window.)
- From the Patient List, select Clarence Hughes (Room 404).
- Click on **Get Report** and read the report.
- Click on **Go to Nurses' Station** and then on **404**.
- Read the **Initial Observations**.
- Click and review **Clinical Alerts**.
- Click on **Chart** and then on **404**.
- Click on and review the **Nurse's Notes** tab.

• Click on **Patient Care** and then on **Nurse-Client Interactions**.
   • Select and view video titled 1115: Interventions—Airway. (*Note:* Check the virtual clock to see whether enough time has elapsed. You can use the fast-forward feature to advance the time by 2-minute intervals if the video is not yet available. Then click again on **Patient Care** and **Nurse-Client Interactions** to refresh the screen.)

   1. What is the primary teaching need for Clarence Hughes at this time?
      a. Physical limitations after discharge
      b. The pathophysiology of the respiratory complications being experienced
      c. The immediate plan of care
      d. The location of the physician

   2. What changes have taken place in Clarence Hughes' condition?

   3. Discuss the need to change the teaching plans in relation to the recent turn of events.

   4. What factors will be used to determine the amount of information that should be presented about Clarence Hughes and his family at this time?

➤ • Click on and review the **Physician's Orders** tab for this period of care.

5. What new physician orders have been added in response to the presentation of complications?

6. Which of the following topics represents the most important teaching needs of Clarence Hughes at this time?
   a. Knowledge of the pathophysiology of the pulmonary complications being experienced
   b. Information concerning prognosis for the client who has a pulmonary embolus
   c. Risk factors for the development of a pulmonary embolus
   d. Knowledge of the immediate treatment plan to manage the pulmonary complications

7. When determining the primary teaching needs for Clarence Hughes, what factors should be considered? Select all that apply.

   _____ Date of planned discharge

   _____ Age of the client

   _____ Cognitive level of the client

   _____ Current physical condition

   _____ Psychological needs

   _____ Prescribed plan of care

8. During a clinical emergency in which a client is unable to provide written or verbal consent, how does the health care team determine the wishes of the client?

9. Develop two nursing diagnoses that reflect the current needs of Clarence Hughes.

10. What impact will the stressors of Clarence Hughes' condition and its emergent nature have on his ability to receive effective client education?

11. When will Clarence Hughes be able to resume discussion concerning the plans for discharge?

LESSON 9 ─────────────────────────

Growth and Development: Infancy to Young Adulthood

───────────────────────────────────────

 Reading Assignment: Infancy Through School-Age Development (Chapter 16)
The Adolescent and Young Adult (Chapter 17)

Client: Dorothy Grant, Obstetrics Floor, Room 201

Objectives:

1. Compare and contrast significant theories of growth and development.
2. Identify developmental milestones and tasks.
3. Describe environmental, socioeconomic, nutritional, and physiological factors affecting growth and development.
4. Describe the assessment of growth and development and health maintenance.
5. Plan interventions to promote growth and development and health maintenance activities.

Exercise 1

 Clinical Preparation: Writing Activity

🕐 15 minutes

1. The physiological development of a living being and the qualitative changes seen in the

   body are known as _____.

2. _____ is the progression of behavioral changes that involve the acquisi-
   tion of appropriate cognitive, linguistic, and psychosocial skills.

3. Neuromuscular growth and development takes place in a _____ manner.

4. Proximodistal development begins at the _____ of the body and moves
   outward.

5. Match each of the following developmental milestones with the average age of its achievement. (*Note:* Some age groups will have more milestones than others.)

Developmental Milestone	Age of Achievement
_____ Sits with support	a. 0 to 1 month
_____ Screws and unscrews jar lids	b. 1 to 3 months
_____ Holds a writing instrument	c. 4 to 7 months
_____ Finds hidden objects	d. 8 to 12 months
_____ Brings hand to mouth	e. 1 to 2 years
_____ Differentiates between light and dark	f. 2 to 3 years
_____ Begins hand-eye coordination	
_____ Responds to touch	
_____ Drinks from a cup	
_____ Sorts objects	

6. While caring for a male child, the nurse notes the child demonstrates behaviors that indicate he is able to understand the thinking and behaviors of others. Based on your knowledge, the child is demonstrating which of the following developmentally appropriate behaviors?
   a. Conservation
   b. Observation
   c. Subjective thinking
   d. Concrete operations

7. When providing health education to a preteen female, the nurse should incorporate which of the following characteristics into the presentation?
   a. The rate of physical growth exceeds the rate of cognitive development.
   b. If the child has begun to demonstrate physical changes, she is considered to be an adolescent.
   c. Some girls in this age group may begin to demonstrate the changes associated with puberty.
   d. The rate of physical growth exceeds the rate of psychosocial development.

8. Indicate whether each of the following statements is true or false.

   a. _____ The growth of the brain is complete around the age of 15.

   b. _____ Adequacy of financial resources can impact parenting skills.

9. The parents of two young children question the nurse about the dangers of lead poisoning. Which of the following statements is correct and should be considered by the nurse when formulating a response? Select all that apply.

_____ Lead poisoning is not a concern in rural communities.

_____ The risk for lead poisoning is greater in Caucasian children than in African-American children.

_____ Children from families who are socioeconomically challenged are at the greatest risk for development of lead poisoning.

_____ Lead poisoning can be fatal.

_____ The damage caused by lead poisoning can be easily reversed.

10. _____ of _____ is defined as an absence of early signs of puberty.

11. Gynecomastia is a serious disorder that normally requires hormonal therapies to resolve.
    a. True
    b. False

Exercise 2

CD-ROM Activity

30 minutes

- Sign in to work at Pacific View Regional Hospital on the Obstetrics Floor for Period of Care 2. (*Note:* If you are already in the virtual hospital from a previous exercise, click on **Leave the Floor** and then **Restart the Program** to get to the sign-in window.)
- From the Patient List, select Dorothy Grant (Room 201).
- Click on **Get Report** and read the report.
- Click on **Go to Nurses' Station** and then on **201** at the bottom of the screen.
- Click on and review the **Clinical Alerts**.
- Click on **Chart** and then on **201**.
- Click on and review the **Nursing Admission**, **History and Physical**, and **Physician's Notes** tabs.

1. Why has Dorothy Grant sought medical care?

2. Dorothy Grant is presently in the stage of _____.

3. The nurse is preparing to develop a plan of care for Dorothy Grant. Which of Erikson's stages of development applies to the client?
   a. Trust versus mistrust
   b. Identity versus role confusion
   c. Generativity versus stagnation
   d. Ego integrity versus despair
   e. Intimacy versus isolation

4. The presence of egocentrism in Dorothy Grant's behaviors would indicate successful transition through the age-appropriate stage of development.
   a. True
   b. False

5. Which of the following tasks much be completed for successful achievement of the Erikson developmental stage that applies to Dorothy Grant? Select all that apply.

   _____   Avoidance of marriage

   _____   Nurturing of successful relationships with a significant other

   _____   Self-acceptance

   _____   Providing of service to community agencies

   _____   Beginning to act in a caretaker relationship with aging parents

• Click on and review the **Nurse's Notes** tab.

6. What behaviors and concerns reported in the Nurse's Notes demonstrate consistency with the tasks of Erikson's stage of development for Dorothy Grant? Why?

7. Which of the following behaviors would demonstrate unsuccessful passage through the age-appropriate Erikson stage of development for Dorothy Grant?
   a. Mistrust of friends and family
   b. Inability to consider the viewpoints of others
   c. Inability to establish relationships with others
   d. The decision not to have children

8. Discuss the current life factors that are interrupting Dorothy Grant's ability to successfully complete the age-appropriate Erikson developmental stage.

9. According to Levinson's Developmental Phases for the Young Adult, which of the following tasks are currently being managed by Dorothy Grant? Select all that apply.

_____ Meeting the transition between adolescence and the adult world

_____ A vision of the future

_____ Realization of dependency on others

_____ Building an initial life structure

_____ A time of exploration

→ • Click on **Chart** and then on **201**.
  • Click on and review the **Consultations** tab.

10. What consultations have been ordered for Dorothy Grant?

11. What are her primary psychosocial concerns at this time?

→ • Click on and review the **Nursing Admission** tab.

12. What is Dorothy Grant's primary physical concern at this time?

13. According to the Nursing Admission, how does Dorothy Grant feel about her current pregnancy? (*Hint:* See page 5 of the report.)

LESSON 10

Growth and Development: Middle to Older Adulthood

Reading Assignment: The Middle and Older Adult (Chapter 18)

Client: Kathryn Doyle, Skilled Nursing Floor, Room 503

Objectives:

1. Compare and contrast significant theories of growth and development.
2. Identify developmental milestones and tasks.
3. Describe environmental, socioeconomic, nutritional, and physiological factors affecting growth and development.
4. Describe the assessment of growth and development and health maintenance.
5. Plan interventions to promote growth and development and health maintenance activities.

Exercise 1

Clinical Preparation: Writing Activity

15 minutes

1. _Geriatric_ nursing is a division of nursing dealing with the problems and diseases of old age and aging people.

2. The process of gradual change in the physical, mental, social, and emotional self resulting in maturation by the mid-20s and followed by a gradual decline into old age and death is

   known as _aging_ .

3. Identify the phases of adulthood, according to the textbook. (*Hint:* See pages 350 and 371 in your textbook).

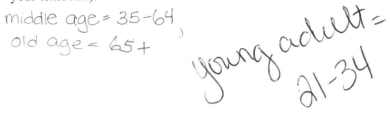

middle age = 35-64,
old age = 65+

young adult = 21-34

4. The fastest growing segment of the U.S. population is the middle adult age group.
   a. True
   b. False   over 85

5. Match each of the following theories of aging with its correct description.

Theory	Description
c Seasons of life	a. Supports the belief that older adults gradually withdraw from social roles in response to declining abilities
a Disengagement	
e Activity	b. A biological theory that the body acts in response to chemical stimuli
f Continuity	
b Free-radical	c. Emphasizes the view of adult life having continuous, distinct eras
d Genetic	d. Promotes the understanding that the aging process is determined by hereditary factors
	e. Advocates that successful aging is a response to maintaining social activities
	f. Supports the belief that aging is determined by the individual's ability to adapt to life changes

6. List the lifestyle risk factors that play a role in the success of the aging process. (*Hint:* See pages 374-375 in your textbook.)

Diet
Exercise
Rest & Sleep
Stress
Risky behaviors (smoking, alcohol abuse, illicit drug use)

7. ___Ageism___ is a stereotype, prejudice, or discrimination against people, especially older adults based on their age.

8. The leading cause of death for older adults is:
   a. Heart disease
   b. Unintentional injuries
   c. AIDS
   d. Bone cancer

9. Indicate whether each of the following statements is true or false.

   a. ___True___ The prevalence of diabetes among Hispanics is greater than for white Americans. *also A.A, N.A., Native Alaskans*

   b. ___False___ Some degree of confusion is a normal part of aging.

10. Match each of the developmental tasks below with the age range in which it occurs, as defined by Levinson's theory on aging.

Levinson's Developmental Task	Age Range
___c___ Stable period of fulfillment	a. 38-42
___a___ Recognition of no longer being young	b. 44-46
___b___ Restabilization	c. 47-59
___e___ Beginning to prepare for death	d. 60-65
___b___ Midlife transition	e. 65-death
___b___ Fullest and most creative period of life	
___d___ Work is no longer the central focus	
___d___ Beginning to spend more time pursuing personal interests	

Exercise 2

 CD-ROM Activity

 30 minutes

- Sign in to work at Pacific View Regional Hospital on the Skilled Nursing Floor for Period Care 2. (*Note:* If you are already in the virtual hospital from a previous exercise, click on **Leave the Floor** and then **Restart the Program** to get to the sign-in window.)
- From the Patient List, select Kathryn Doyle (Room 503).
- Click on **Get Report** and read the **Clinical Report**.
- Click on **Go to Nurses' Station** and then on **503** at the bottom of the screen.
- Click on **Check Armband** and then on **Take Vital Signs**. Review the information given.

1. How old is Kathryn Doyle?

79

2. At Kathryn Doyle's current age, ___*7–8*___ hours of sleep each night are recommended for her.

3. In what phase of adulthood is Kathryn Doyle?

Old age

4. Which Erikson stage of development is applicable to Karen Doyle?
   a. Trust versus mistrust
   b. Ego Integrity versus despair
   c. Generativity versus stagnation
   d. Identity versus identity confusion

pg 351a table 18-1 *usually youngest stage*

5. Which of the following developmental tasks face Kathryn Doyle during this phase of her life? Select all that apply.

   ___✓___ Reflection on one's own mortality

   _____ Interest in community activities

   _____ Longing to participate in civic matters

   ___✓___ Acceptance of one's own death

   _____ Beginning to share duties with one's life partner

6. According to Levinson's development phases, Kathryn Doyle is in a stable period of fulfill-ment.
   a. True
   b. False   *If not, will despair + fear death*

• Click on **Chart** and then on **503**.
• Click on and review the **Nursing Admission** tab.

7. Why has Kathryn Doyle been admitted to the Skilled Nursing Unit?

Complicated Recovery from ORIF

broke hip when getting out of bed.

→ • Click on **Return to Room 503**.
  • Click on **Patient Care** and then on **Physical Assessment**.
  • Complete a head-to-toe assessment.

8. What age-related changes are noted in Kathryn Doyle's skin?

↓ turgor *dry, coarse, thin hair*
lentigens
Thin
dry

9. Identify any other significant age-related changes in Kathryn Doyle's assessment.

denture, ↓cognition, ↓ROM
crackles in lower lobes
weakness + unsteady gait
Stress incontinence (more common
in women)

→ • Click on **MAR** and review the medications ordered for Kathryn Doyle.

10. Which of the following statements are true concerning the use of medications in older adults? Select all that apply.

✓ On average, the older adult takes up to seven prescription medications.

✓ Laxatives and vitamin supplements are commonly used medications among older adults.

___ The average older adult is currently taking only two prescription medications.

___ The use of multiple drugs will enhance the therapeutic benefits of the medications taken.

✓ Using more than one pharmacy to fill prescriptions will increase risk factors associated with polypharmacy.

___ The body's ability to absorb, transport, and eliminate mediations is increased with age.

→ • Click on **Return to Room 503**.
  • Click on the **Drug** icon to access the Drug Guide. Read about the medications ordered for Kathryn Doyle.

11. Which of the ordered medications listed below have special lifespan considerations listed for older adults? Select all that apply.

   ___✓___ Calcium citrate

   _____ Ferrous sulfate

   _____ Docusate sodium

   ___✓___ Ibuprofen

   ___✓___ Oxycodone

   _____ Acetaminophen

12. Identify steps that can reduce medication-related complications in the older client.

Teach about interactions of prescribed + OTC drugs

Teach them to drink plenty of fluids

Explaing aging ↓ absorption + ↓ kidney function causes ↓ in amount excreted

Carry complete list of meds

Make sure clients are aware of their allergies + to comm. them to HCP.

LESSON **11**

Health Perception

 Reading Assignment: Health Perception (Chapter 19)
Health Maintenance: Lifestyle Management (Chapter 20)

Clients: Harry George, Medical-Surgical Floor, Room 401
Jacquline Catanazaro, Medical-Surgical Floor, Room 402
Patricia Newman, Medical-Surgical Floor, Room 406

Objectives:

1. Describe the perception of health for individuals, families, and communities.
2. Identify factors that affect health for individuals, families, and communities.
3. Identify methodologies of intervention for improving the health of individuals, families, and communities.
4. Describe factors affecting behavorial change.
5. Assess the client experiencing problems maintaining health when a therapeutic regimen requires alterations in lifestyle.

Exercise 1

Clinical Preparation: Writing Activity

30 minutes

1. _____ is the knowledge and experience of one's state of wellness and well-being.

2. _____ refers to the advancement of health through activities that enhance wellness.

3. Identify the five interrelating factors that affect health. (*Hint:* See pages 399-400 in your textbook.)

4. When collecting data concerning individual health patterns, which of the following questions and or statements by the nurse would be most effective?
   a. Do you enjoy your job?
   b. Would you rate your coping skills as adequate?
   c. Describe your family's interpersonal relationships.
   d. Discuss methods you use to cope during times of stress and illness.

5. Health is a static condition.
   a. True
   b. False

6. Match each activity below with its corresponding level of prevention. (*Hint:* Each of the levels can be used more than once.)

Activity	**Level of Prevention**
_____ A 41-year-old woman seeks an annual mammogram.	a. Primary prevention
_____ The nurse provides a class discussing the importance of breast self-examination.	b. Secondary prevention
	c. Tertiary prevention
_____ A client who has been critically injured in an accident undergoes occupational therapy.	
_____ A client attends a preconception class offered by the local hospital.	

7. The objective interpretation of health by a scientifically trained practitioner is known as

_____.

8. Which of the following statements are correct about the Western worldview? Select all that apply.

_____ Emphasizes group cooperation

_____ Emphasizes task orientation

_____ Values achievement for the individual

_____ Adheres to a rigid time schedule

_____ Sees time as relative

_____ Thinks holistically

_____ Prefers nuclear family

9. Western medicine uses a _____, _____, and

_____ approach to explain illness.

Exercise 2

 CD-ROM Activity

 15 minutes

- Sign in to work at Pacific View Regional Hospital on Medical-Surgical Floor for Period of Care 1. (*Note:* If you are already in the virtual hospital from a previous exercise, click on **Leave the Floor** and then **Restart the Program** to get to the sign-in window.)
- From the Patient List, select Jacquline Catanazaro (Room 402).
- Click on **Get Report** and read the report.
- Click on **Go to Nurses' Station**.
- Click on **Chart** and then on **402**.
- Click on and review the **Nursing Admission** tab.

1. What are Jacquline Catanazaro's diagnoses?

2. Based on your review of the Nursing Admission data, complete the following dietary history.

Height

Weight

History of food allergies

Number of meals per day

Food preferences

Food preparation practices

Appetite

History of weight change

Condition of oral cavity

Bowel elimination

3. Explain how Jacquline Catanazaro's obesity affects her ability to breathe.

4. How does Jacquline Catanazaro describe her pattern of activity?

5. Which of the following factors contribute to Jacquline Catanazaro's bowel elimination problems? Select all that apply.

_____ Physical inactivity

_____ Age

_____ Emotional stress

_____ Limited intake of high-fiber foods

_____ Reduced fluid intake

_____ Obesity

6. Jacquline Catanazaro reportedly can become very anxious because of her mental illness. Which of the following best describes the influence anxiety has on the client's oxygenation status?
   a. Causes hypoventilation
   b. Increases the body's metabolic rate and oxygen demand
   c. Reduces the diffusion of oxygen across the alveolar membrane
   d. Creates a sense of breathlessness from CO2 retention

7. Jacquline Catanazaro's medical conditions are not well-controlled because of her noncompliance with medication therapies. What does she state as the reason for her noncompliance?

8. How does Jacquline Catanazaro feel that her medical problems have affected her lifestyle?

9. Explain the interrelationships among Jacquline Catanazaro's medical conditions and the negative effects that her lifestyle choices can have on her health.

Exercise 3

 CD-ROM Activity

 15 minutes

• Sign in to work at Pacific View Regional Hospital on the Medical-Surgical Floor for Period of Care 2. (*Note:* If you are already in the virtual hospital from a previous exercise, click on **Leave the Floor** and then **Restart the Program** to get to the sign-in window.)

• From the Patient List, select Patricia Newman (Room 406).

• Click on **Get Report** and read the report.

• Click on **Go to Nurses' Station**.

• Click on **Chart** and then on **406**.

• Click on and review the **Nursing Admission** and **History and Physical**.

1. Patricia Newman has a history of emphysema and hypertension. What is one factor in her history that could be associated with both conditions?

2. The client's statement describing her health as "not very good" is an example of:
   a. objective data.
   b. back channeling.
   c. defining character.
   d. subjective data.

3. Patricia Newman is 61 years old. Let's assume that she has smoked since the age of 22. If so, how many packs of cigarettes would she have averaged on a daily basis? (*Hint:* Apply the formula for pack-year history in your textbook.)

4. Based on the information you have reviewed so far, list four learning needs that apply to Patricia Newman.

5. List three lifestyle risk factors that likely contribute to Patricia Newman's emphysema and hypertension.

6. Patricia Newman's history reveals poor adherence to health promotion behaviors. As her nurse, what recommendations might you make to prevent future occurrences of pneumonia?

7. Explain the interrelationships among Patricia Newman's medical conditions and the negative effects that her lifestyle choices can have on her health.

Exercise 4

 CD-ROM Activity

 15 minutes

- Sign in to work at Pacific View Regional Hospital on the Medical-Surgical Floor for Period of Care 3. (*Note:* If you are already in the virtual hospital from a previous exercise, click on **Leave the Floor** and then **Restart the Program** to get to the sign-in window.)
- From the Patient List, select Harry George (Room 401).
- Click on **Get Report** and read the report.
- Click on **Go to Nurses' Station**.
- Click on **Chart** and then on 401.
- Click on and review the **Nursing Admission** tab.
- Click on the **Consultations** tab and review the Psychiatric Consult.
- Click on and review the Mental Health tab.

1. What does Harry George give as his reasons for hospitalization?

2. Complete the table below by providing data for each category based on your review of the Nursing Admission for Harry George.

Reason for admission/
chief complaint

Nutrition/
Metabolic

Skin

Activity/Rest

Self-Perception

Pain

3. Listed below are factors that influence wound healing. Place an X next to all of the factors that apply to Harry George.

_____ Nutrition

_____ Smoking

_____ Circulation

_____ Drugs

_____ Obesity

_____ Infection

_____ Age

_____ Wound stress

_____ Diabetes

4. What factor(s) in Harry George's social history may be implicated in his ability to care for his wound? Explain.

5. A focused assessment will help the nurse better understand the nature of the stress affecting Harry George. For each of the assessment categories below, write two questions you would ask this client.

Perception of stressor

Adherence to healthy practices

6. As the nurse, you review the Activity/Rest portion of the Nursing Admission history. Harry George's sleep pattern is documented as being "irregular, never more than 2 hours." You decide to question the client further about the sleep habits he follows—the time he normally goes to bed, activities prior to going to sleep, and number of awakenings during night. Your decision is an example of what critical thinking attitude?
   a. Humility
   b. Thinking independently
   c. Risk taking
   d. Perseverance

7. Explain the interrelationships among Harry George's medical conditions and the negative effects that his lifestyle choices can have on his health.

LESSON 12

Medication Management

Reading Assignment: Health Maintenance: Medication Management (Chapter 21)

Client: Piya Jordan, Medical-Surgical Floor, Room 403

Objectives:

1. Identify important concepts related to safe and effective medication management.
2. Describe a variety of factors that influence drug actions in individual clients.
3. Explain how to assess a client who is receiving medication therapy.
4. Incorporate safe and effective nursing interventions in the care of a client receiving medications.
5. Evaluate the effectiveness of medication therapy in helping to achieve health-related expected outcomes.

131

Exercise 1

Clinical Preparation: Writing Activity

30 minutes

1. Match each of the following key terms with its correct definition.

Key Term	Definition
_b_ Chemical name	a. Amount of medication available for use by target tissues
_d_ Generic name	b. A precise description of the components and structure of a medication
_c_ Trade name	c. The copyrighted name for a medication given by a specific manufacturer
_e_ Classification	d. The nonproprietary name assigned to a drug by the United States Adopted Names Council
_a_ Bioavailability	e. Groupings of medications having shared actions
_f_ OTC medication	f. Medications available without a prescription from a physician
_g_ Official name	g. The name assigned to a drug by the Food and Drug Administration after it is approved for use

2. Which of the following government agencies has the authority to enforce narcotic laws?
    a. The U.S. Adopted Names Council
    b. The Food and Drug Administration
    (c.) The Drug Enforcement Agency
    d. The American Hospital Formulary Service

3. A _prescription_ is an order for a medication that details the client's name, medication name, and dosing information.

4. A client exhibits a rash after the administration of an antibiotic. Since the client has successfully taken the medication in the past, it is not possible that the rash is an allergic reaction to the antibiotic.
    a. True
    (b.) False

5. A client is exhibiting symptoms consistent with anaphylaxis. Which of the following manifestations would be anticipated? Select all that apply.

    _____ Nausea

    _____ Bradycardia

    _____ Tachycardia

    _____ Hypotension

_____ Hypertension

✓ Wheezing

✓ Rhonchi in the lower lung lobes

6. The toxic effects of a medication may be reversed with a(n) _antidote_.

7. An allergic response to a medication is the result of a(n) _antibody_ - _antigen_ response.

8. When preparing to administer medications to a client, the Six Rights of administration must be reviewed. List these rights.

    Right patient
    Right dose
    Right time
    Right drug
    Right Route
    Right documentation

9. When the nurse is providing education to a client regarding recognition of individual medications, color is a good guide to use.
   a. True
   b. False

10. To ensure that medication reaches the stomach and does not stick in the esophagus, it is best to encourage the client to drink at least _60_ to _100_ mL of fluid with the final tablet taken.
    50 - 60mL in workbook

11. Which of the following types of medications cannot be crushed? Select all that apply.

    ✓ Enteric-coated

    ✓ Extended-action

    ✓ Sublingual

    ✓ Buccal

12. The _gauge_ of a needle refers to its diameter.

13. Which of the following medication administration situations require that a larger-gauge needle be used? Select all that apply. (*Hint:* See page 459 in your textbook.)

_____ The client is underweight.

_____ The client is a male.

✓ Larger volumes of medications are being administered.

✓ The medication is viscous.

✓ The medication must penetrate to deeper tissues.

14. Indicate whether each of the following statements is true or false.

a. _True___ After the medication has been withdrawn from a vial, changing the needle will reduce tissue irritation by the client.

b. _True___ The absorption rate for subcutaneous administration of medication is prolonged.

15. An intradermal administration requires the needle to be inserted bevel-up at an angle of __~~5~~ to _15_ degrees.
? . 10 - 15

Exercise 2

 CD-ROM Activity

🕐 45 minutes

- Sign in to work at Pacific View Regional Hospital on the Medical-Surgical Floor for Period of Care 1. (*Note:* If you are already in the virtual hospital from a previous exercise, click on **Leave the Floor** and then **Restart the Program** to get to the sign-in window.)
- From the Patient List, select Piya Jordan (Room 403).
- Click on **Get Report** and read the report.
- Click on **Go to Nurses' Station** and then on **403**.
- Read the **Initial Observations**.
- Click on **Clinical Alerts** and read the information given.

1. Identify the behavioral manifestations in Piya Jordan that warrant further evaluation.

AM- Patient confused, Restless, agitated —check airway, breathing, circulation first!!

Pulling @ tubes & IV

* Oriented to person only

2. The suspected cause of Piya Jordan's disorientation is:
   a. morphine toxicity.
   b. elevated potassium level.
   c. low serum potassium level.
   d. meperidine toxicity. *(circled)*

3. Identify the clinical manifestations associated with the problem you identified in question 2. Select all that apply. (*Hint:* You can use the Drug Guide to find this information.)

   _____ Tachycardia

   ___✓___ Respiratory depression

   _____ Warm, flushed skin

   ___✓___ Convulsions

   ___✓___ Stupor

   ___✓___ Skeletal muscle flaccidity

→ • Click on **Patient Care** and then on **Nurse-Client Interactions**.
   • Select and view the video titled **0735: Pain—Adverse Drug Event**. (*Note:* Check the virtual clock to see whether enough time has elapsed. You can use the fast-forward feature to advance the time by 2-minute intervals if the video is not yet available. Then click again on **Patient Care** and **Nurse-Client Interactions** to refresh the screen.)
   • Click on **Chart** and then on **403**.
   • Click on and review the **Physician's Orders**, **Physician's Notes**, and **Nurse's Notes** tabs.

4. To which factors can Piya Jordan's meperidine toxicity be attributed? Select all that apply.

   ___✓___ Advancing age

   (scribbled out) Gastrointestinal malignancy

   Impaired liver function

   ___✓___ Her daughter's misuse of the PCA pump controls

5. What changes in analgesics have been ordered by the physician?

   Discontinue Meperidine
   Change PCA to morphine
   Sulfate 1mg/mL

6. The physician's order to change Piya Jordan's analgesics can best be classified as a:
   a. prn order.
   b. standing order. *(circled)*
   c. single order.
   d. stat order.

7. Piya Jordan's analgesic is being administered via PCA pump. What do the initials PCA stand for?

Patient Controlled Analgesia

8. When assessing Piya Jordan's vital signs before and during the administration of morphine, the nurse should use which of the following as a critical indicator of whether the medication can be administered?
   a. Heart rate
   b. Respiratory rate *(circled)*
   c. Temperature
   d. Blood pressure

9. Morphine is a Schedule II narcotic. Which of the following statements best explains this classification?
   a. The drug has medically acceptable uses with minimal risk for abuse or dependence.
   b. The agent is not readily accepted for medical use because of its high potential for abuse.
   c. The medication has acceptable medical uses with limited risk for abuse or dependence.
   d. The substance has acceptable medical uses but also has a high potential for abuse or physical or psychological dependency. *(circled)*

→ • Click on **MAR** and review Piya Jordan's ordered morphine PCA dosages.

10. Are these dosages within recommended ranges? (*Hint:* Refer to the Drug Guide to review recommended dosages.)

1mg q 10 min/ 2mg/ 4-hr lockout IV continuous - 30 mL prefilled syringe
Yes

11. The physician has ordered "no loading dose" for Piya Jordan's PCA administration. What is a loading dose?

An initial dose

12. _Toxicity Reactions_ are serious adverse effects of medications that may threaten life.

13. Piya Jordan's potassium level is _3.4_ mEq/L.

14. When will Piya Jordan's potassium levels be reassessed?

15. The normal range for potassium level is between _3.5_ and _5.0_ mEq/L.

16. Piya Jordan has reduced levels of potassium. This is known as:
    a. hypocalcemia.
    b. hypercalcemia.
    c. hyperkalemia.
    d. hypokalemia.

17. The physician has ordered 20 mEq of potassium chloride to be given IV. When is this medication dosage scheduled to be repeated?
    a. Not scheduled to be repeated
    b. Tomorrow morning at the same time
    c. In 12 hours
    d. After the 1800 serum potassium levels are checked

    —to infuse over 2hr.

18. Match each of the following ordered medications with its correct classification.

	Medication		Classification
C	Morphine	a.	Antiemetic
a	Ondansetron	b.	Antibiotic
d	Enoxaparin	c.	Analgesic
e	Promethazine	d.	Anticoagulant
b	Cefotan	e.	Sedative-hypnotic

19. Piya Jordan has an order for enoxaparin by subcutaneous administration. After administering the medication, is it appropriate to rub the site? Why or why not?

    No, b/c it will cause faster absorption

20. When the nurse administers enoxaparin, a ____ to ____-gauge and ____ to ____-inch needle should be used.

21. Prior to administration of enoxaparin, which of the following test results should be reviewed?
    a. Complete blood cell count
    b. Urinalysis
    c. Chest x-ray
    d. ECG

LESSON 13

Medication Administration

 Reading Assignment: Health Maintenance: Medication Management (Chapter 21)

Clients: Piya Jordan, Medical-Surgical Floor, Room 403
Kathryn Doyle, Skilled Nursing Floor, Room 503

Objectives:

1. Discuss the rationale for medications ordered for clients in case studies.
2. Explain how to apply the Six Rights of medication administration.
3. Perform medication dosage calculations.
4. Explain nursing implications for administering medications.
5. Describe potential sources of medication errors.
6. Identify factors that influence selection of form and route of a medication for administration.
7. Discuss factors in the case studies that would contraindicate administration of a medication.
8. Correctly describe steps for administering a medication.

Medication administration is one of the more important responsibilities of a professional nurse because of the risks involved. Any given medication has the potential for creating harmful effects if administered inappropriately or incorrectly. The busy health care environment poses many barriers to safe medication administration. Thus it is important to learn how to attend to the preparation and administration of medications. You can never be too cautious in administering medications. Always follow the Six Rights of drug administration and be aware of the principles used to calculate and prepare medications safely and accurately. Know the effects that medications may have on your client's behavior and physical condition so that you can properly monitor the client and evaluate whether the drugs have been effective.

Client education is an important part of drug therapy. Clients must obtain the necessary information to self-administer medications safely and know how to monitor their response to medications. Home environments and daily routines influence how clients take their medications. It is important to problem-solve with clients and families to anticipate possible barriers to safe medication administration in the home and workplace.

Exercise 1

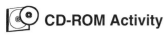

CD-ROM Activity

45 minutes

In this exercise you will visit Piya Jordan, a 68-year-old Asian-American female who entered the hospital after an Emergency Department admission for abdominal pain, nausea, and vomiting. She underwent abdominal surgery for the removal of a mass in her right lower quadrant.

- Sign in to work at Pacific View Regional Hospital on the Medical-Surgical Floor for Period of Care 1. (*Note:* If you are already in the virtual hospital from a previous exercise, click on **Leave the Floor** and then **Restart the Program** to get to the sign-in window.)
- From the Patient List, select Piya Jordan (Room 403).
- Click on **Get Report** and review the report.
- Click on **Go to Nurses' Station**.
- Click on **Chart** and then on **403**.
- Review the **History and Physical**.
- Next, review the **Physician's Orders** for Tuesday and Wednesday mornings.

1. Piya Jordan has orders for a number of medications postoperatively. Match each medication listed below with the rationale for its administration.

Medication	Rationale
_____ Digoxin 0.125 mg IV	a. Reduce fever
_____ Famotidine 20 mg IV	b. Reduce gastric acid secretion
_____ Cefotetan 1 g IV	c. Slow the heart rate (atrial fibrillation)
_____ Acetaminophen 650 mg per rectum q6h	d. Prevent postop wound infection

2. Review the physician's postop medication orders once again. Are there any dangerous abbreviations used? If so, what is the preferred alternative?

• Once again, review the physician's medication orders for Piya Jordan.
- Now click on **Return to Nurses' Station**.
- Click on the **Medication Room**.
- Select the **MAR** and click tab **403**.
- Review the MAR for drugs due to be given to Piya Jordan on Wednesday between 0730 and 0815.

3. Place an X next to all of the following statements that describe activities for correctly following the Six Rights of medication administration.

_____ Compare MAR with physician's written order for the name of a medication.

_____ Review the medical record for the client's allergies.

_____ Review the supply cart for the size of syringes.

_____ Check the MAR against the physician's written order for the route to give a medication.

_____ Compare the physician's written order for a medication with the times selected on the MAR for scheduled administration.

 • Click on **Return to Medication Room**.
- Based on your care for Piya Jordan, access the various storage areas of the Medication Room to obtain the necessary medications you need to administer.
- For each area you access, select the medication you plan to administer and then click **Put Medication on Tray**. When finished with a storage area, click on **Close Drawer** or **Close Bin**.
- Click **View Medication Room**.
- Now click on **Preparation** and choose the correct medication to administer. Click **Prepare**.
- Click **Next** and choose the correct client to administer this medication to. Click **Finish**.
- You can **Review Your Medications** and then **Return to Medication Room** when ready.

4. How much of the digoxin did you prepare in a syringe for Piya Jordan?

5. Which of the following medications did you prepare for this time period? Select all that apply.

_____ Enoxaparin 40 mg

_____ KCl 20 mEq in 250 mL NS

_____ Digoxin 0.125 mg

_____ Morphine sulfate 2.5 mg per 1 mL

_____ Cefotetan 1 g

• Click on **Return to Nurses' Station**.
   • Click on **403** at the bottom of the screen.

6. Before administering digoxin to Piya Jordan, what should you assess?
   a. Blood pressure and IV infusion
   b. Apical heart rate and IV infusion
   c. Potassium level and blood pressure
   d. Client's level of discomfort and range of motion in knees

7. Before you administer the digoxin, what is the main function of the IV infusion you should assess?

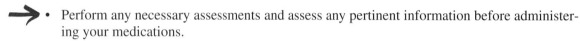 • Perform any necessary assessments and assess any pertinent information before administering your medications.
   • After you have collected the appropriate assessment data and are ready for administration, click **Patient Care** and **Medication Administration**. Verify that the correct client and medication(s) appear in the left-hand window. Then click the down arrow next to Select. From the drop-down menu, select **Administer** and complete the Administration Wizard by providing any information requested. When the Wizard stops asking for information, click **Administer to Patient**. Specify **Yes** when asked whether this administration should be recorded in the MAR. Finally, click **Finish**.

8. Indicate whether each of the following statements is true or false.

   a. _____ IV administration of digoxin creates a greater risk to the client than IV administration of KCl.

   b. _____ After choosing to hold cefotetan because of Piya Jordan's allergy, you should contact the prescriber immediately.

   c. _____ When you are administering a medication by an intermittent infusion, you should turn off the main IV infusion as the medication is infused.

   d. _____ After administering an intermittent infusion, you should discard the bag of medication and the IV tubing.

9. Why is Piya Jordan not given her digoxin by mouth?

Exercise 2

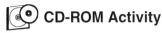 **CD-ROM Activity**

 45 minutes

- Sign in to work at Pacific View Regional Hospital on the Medical-Surgical Floor for Period of Care 2. (*Note:* If you are already in the virtual hospital from a previous exercise, click on **Leave the Floor** and then **Restart the Program** to get to the sign-in window.)
- From the Patient List, select Piya Jordan (Room 403).
- Click on **Get Report** and review the report.
- Click on **Go to Nurses' Station**.
- Click on **Chart** and then on **403**.
- Review the **History and Physical**.
- Then select **Nurse's Notes** and review.
- Next, review the **Physician's Orders**.

1. The physician ordered ondansetron 4 mg IV q6h PRN for nausea. Which of the following statements are true about a PRN order?

   _____ It calls for a single dose of a medication to be given only once.

   _____ It is a type of order that requires the medication to be given at a specific time.

   _____ It is an order prescribed for a time when a client requires the medication.

   _____ It is the only type of order canceled when a client goes to surgery.

The physician also ordered enoxaparin 40 mg SubQ. Fill in the blanks below to describe principles for administering subcutaneous injections.

2. A subcutaneous injection requires a _____-gauge needle

3. A _____ to _____-mL syringe is usually adequate for a subcutaneous injection.

4. The best site for administering heparin is the _____.

5. Injecting heparin slowly over 30 seconds may create less _____.

6. Considering Piya Jordan's physical build, what needle length and angle of insertion would you use for the enoxaparin injection?

• Click on **Return to Nurses' Station**.
 • Click on **403** at the bottom of the screen.
 • Review the **Initial Observations**.
 • Click on **Patient Care** and then on **Nurse-Client Interactions**.
 • Select and view the video titled **1115: Interventions—Nausea, Blood**. (*Note:* Check the virtual clock to see whether enough time has elapsed. You can use the fast-forward feature to advance the time by 2-minute intervals if the video is not yet available. Then click again on **Patient Care** and **Nurse-Client Interactions** to refresh the screen.)
 • After viewing the video, click on **Take Vital Signs** at the top of the screen.

   7. Based on your review the physician's medication orders and the video, is it appropriate to administer the ordered acetaminophen for Piya Jordan? Explain.

   8. Piya Jordan has complained of nausea. Go to the Medication Room to prepare ondansetron and then answer the following questions.
      a. The ondansetron comes in a vial/ampule containing how many mL?

      b. What is the correct volume of ondansetron to administer?

 • Click on **Return to Room 403**.
 • Click on **Patient Care** and then on **Physical Assessment**.

9. What body system would you assess prior to administering the ondansetron? Explain your answer.

 • Click on **Medication Room**.

• Click on **MAR** to determine the medications that Piya Jordan is ordered to receive. (*Note:* You may click on **Review MAR** at any time to verify the correct medication order. Remember to look at client name on the MAR to make sure you have the client's record—you must click on the correct room number within the MAR.) Click on **Return to Medication Room** after reviewing the correct MAR.

• Based on your care for Piya Jordan, access the various storage areas of the Medication Room to obtain the necessary medications you need to administer.

• For each area you access, select the medication you plan to administer and then click **Put Medication on Tray**. When finished with a storage area, click on **Close Drawer** or **Close Bin**.

• Click **View Medication Room**.

• Click on **Preparation** and choose the correct medication to administer. Click **Prepare**.

• Click **Next** and choose the correct client to administer this medication to. Click **Finish**.

• You can **Review Your Medications** and then **Return to Medication Room** when ready. Once you are back in the Medication Room, go directly to Piya Jordan's room to administer this medication by clicking on **403** at the bottom of the screen.

• After you have collected the appropriate assessment data and are ready for administration, click **Patient Care** and **Medication Administration**. Verify that the correct client and medication(s) appear in the left-hand window. Then click the down arrow next to Select. From the drop-down menu, select **Administer** and complete the Administration Wizard by providing any information requested. When the Wizard stops asking for information, click **Administer to Patient**. Specify Yes when asked whether this administration should be recorded in the MAR. Finally, click **Finish**.

10. Below is a list of steps describing the proper technique for administering an IV push medication. Indicate the correct sequence by numbering the steps from 1 to 10.

    _____ Clean off injection port with antiseptic swab.

    _____ Recheck fluid infusion rate.

    _____ Perform hand hygiene and apply gloves.

    _____ Select injection port of IV tubing closest to client.

    _____ Check client's identification by looking at identification bracelet and asking client's name.

    _____ Occlude IV line and check for blood return.

    _____ Withdraw syringe from port.

    _____ Connect syringe to IV line.

    _____ Dispose of uncapped needles and syringe and perform hand hygiene.

    _____ Release tubing and inject medication within time recommended.

11. After administering ondansetron, how would you evaluate Piya Jordan for side effects or adverse reactions to the drug?

12. Headache, chest pain, and difficulty breathing can be side effects of ondansetron. If Piya Jordan developed these, what would you do?

13. Checking a client's identification bracelet before administering a medication ensures that you:
    a. administer the medication at the right time.
    b. administer the medication to the right patient.
    c. administer the right medication.
    d. administer the medication with the right documentation.

LESSON 14 ————————————————————

Alterations in Nutrition: Malnutrition

—————————————————————————————————————

Reading Assignment: Promoting Healthy Nutrition (Chapter 24)
Restoring Nutrition (Chapter 25)
Maintaining Fluid and Electrolyte Balance (Chapter 26)

Client: Kathryn Doyle, Skilled Nursing Floor, Room 503

Objectives:

1. Describe elements of a nutritious diet.
2. Identify factors that affect nutritional status.
3. Describe the assessment of a client's nutritional status.
4. Discuss factors that cause nutritional deficits.
5. Assess clients experiencing nutritional deficits.
6. Describe types of electrolytes and their roles in the human body.
7. Describe the general assessment of a client's fluid, electrolyte, and acid-base balance.

Exercise 1

Clinical Preparation: Writing Activity

30 minutes

1. List the five major components of food.

2. Use the MyPyramid food guidance system to match each food group below with the correct number of recommended daily servings. (*Hint:* See the USDA's MyPyramid website: www.mypyramid.gov.)

Food Group	**Number of servings**
_____ Grains	a. 3 cups per day
_____ Vegetables	b. 6 oz per day
_____ Fruits	c. 5½ oz per day
_____ Milk	d. 2 cups per day
_____ Meats and beans	e. 2½ cups per day

3. Major minerals are responsible for the regulation of fluid, _____, and

_____-_____ balance.

 4. List the major minerals needed by the body. (*Hint:* See page 569 in your textbook.)

5. Match each of the following nutrients with the clinical manifestations associated with a deficiency of the nutrient.

Nutrient	**Manifestations of Deficiency**
_____ Vitamin A	a. Retarded bone growth, bone malformation, enlargement of the ends of long bones, malformed teeth, tooth decay
_____ Vitamin C	
_____ Vitamin D	b. Bleeding gums, hemorrhage, muscle degeneration, delayed wound healing
_____ Vitamin E	c. Night blindness, rough dry skin, dry eyes, dry mucous membranes
	d. Possible mild hemolytic anemia in adults, macrocytic anemia in preterm infants

6. Indicate whether each of the following statements is true or false.

   a. _____ Proteins and fiber are called energy nutrients.

   b. _____ Fat should constitute 30% or less of the daily caloric intake.

7. A diet high in fat has been associated with the development of _____,

   _____, and _____.

8. A client has been told to begin taking a multivitamin supplement daily. The client has questions about why this is needed. Which of the following statements is correct?
   a. Vitamins are organic substances.
   b. Vitamins provide energy.
   c. Water-soluble vitamins include the B complexes and vitamin C.
   d. Fat-soluble vitamins cannot be stored in the body.

9. The nurse is providing education to a client concerning the benefits of a high-fiber diet. Which of the following concepts should be included in the exchange of information? Select all that apply.

   _____ Enhanced bowel functioning

   _____ Increased energy

   _____ Reduced blood cholesterol

   _____ Increased rate of glucose absorption

   _____ Reduced incidence of colon cancer development

10. A client has been advised to increase her intake of folic acid in preparation for pregnancy. Which of the following foods should be included in this plan? Select all that apply.

   _____ Milk

   _____ Eggs

   _____ Dried beans

   _____ Whole grain products

   _____ Yeast

   _____ Wheat germ

   _____ Leafy green vegetables

11. While being seen at the physician's office for a routine physical examination, a client tells the nurse he has been hearing a great deal of hype about antioxidants. He asks the nurse to explain what they are. Which of the following statements about antioxidants is most accurate?
    a. Antioxidants are plant pigments found in yellow fruits and vegetables.
    b. Antioxidants are hormone-like substances found in whole grains and legumes.
    c. Antioxidants are contained in some foods and are believed to have a role in the prevention of cancer.
    d. Antioxidants are proteins found in onions and wines and are linked to a reduction in the risk for diabetes.

12. A(n) _____ is any compound that, when dissolved in water, separates into positively charged particles.

13. Match each of the following electrolytes with its correct function in the body.

Electrolyte

_____ Sodium

_____ Potassium

_____ Calcium

_____ Magnesium

_____ Chloride

_____ Phosphate

Function

a. Promotes metabolism of carbohydrates, fats, and proteins; promotes regulation of Ca, PO_4, K

b. Promotes nerve impulse conduction, especially in the heart and skeletal muscles; promotes glycogen storage in the liver

c. Necessary to ATP production; promotes acid-base balance through phosphate buffer system

d. Maintains blood volume; controls water shifting between compartments

e. Promotes blood coagulation; inhibits cell membrane permeability to sodium

f. Inhibits smooth muscle contraction; regulates extracellular fluid volume

Exercise 2

 CD-ROM Activity

 45 minutes

- Sign in to work at Pacific View Regional Hospital on the Skilled Nursing Floor for Period of Care 3. (*Note:* If you are already in the virtual hospital from a previous exercise, click on **Leave the Floor** and then **Restart the Program** to get to the sign-in window.)
- From the Patient List, select Kathryn Doyle (Room 503).
- Click on **Get Report** and read the report.
- Click on **Go to Nurses' Station** and then on **503** to enter the client's room.
- Read the **Initial Observations**.
- Click on **Chart** and then on **503**.
- Click on and review the **History and Physical** and **Nursing Admission** tabs.

1. According to the History and Physical, what is the physician's impression concerning the nutritional status of Kathryn Doyle?

2. Kathryn Doyle weighs 105 pounds and is 64 inches tall. She is approximately _____ pounds under her minimum ideal weight. (*Hint:* See page 574 in your textbook.)

3. The ideal weight, as calculated above, is based on a traditional height-weight table. What are disadvantages of this method?

4. Calculate the body mass index (BMI) for Kathryn Doyle. (*Hint:* See pages 574-575 in your textbook.)

5. Which of the following disease processes are associated with a BMI below the ideal range of 18.5-24.9? Select all that apply.

_____ Diabetes

_____ Respiratory diseases

_____ Digestive diseases

_____ Osteoarthritis

_____ Colon cancer

6. To maintain a healthy body weight, clients must achieve a balance between

_____ and _____.

7. Based on her age, Kathryn Doyle will need approximately _____ calories per day.

8. What complications related to Kathryn Doyle's surgery are reported in the History and Physical?

9. Which of the postoperative complications identified in the previous question are further complicated by Kathryn Doyle's nutritional status? Why does her nutritional status have negative effects on these aspects of her health?

• Click Return to Nurse's Station and then on **503** to enter Kathryn Doyle's room.
• Read the **Initial Observations**.
• Click on **Take Vital Signs** and review the information given.
• Click on **Patient Care** and perform a head-to-toe physical assessment.

10. What assessment findings are related to her limited nutritional intake?

11. What dietary nutrients would aid Kathryn Doyle in increasing her energy level?

→ • Click on **Chart** and then on **503**.
  • Click on and review the **Physician's Orders** tab.

12. According to the physician's orders, Kathryn Doyle is on a _____,

    _____ diet.

→ • Click on and review the **Consultations** tab.

13. Discuss the plan outlined in the Dietary Consultation.

14. Which of the following foods can be included in Kathryn Doyle's ordered diet? Select all that apply.

    _____ Milk

    _____ Tea

    _____ Eggs

    _____ Cabbage

    _____ Whole grain cereal

    _____ Chicken salad

15. Which of the following are risk factors for the development of osteoporosis? Select all that apply.

_____ Female

_____ Male

_____ Caucasian

_____ Hispanic

_____ Steroid use

_____ Cigarette use

_____ Immobility

_____ Inadequate dietary intake

_____ Reduced hormone levels

16. Which of the factors for the development of osteoporosis identified in question 15 are present in Kathryn Doyle?

17. The recommended daily amount of calcium intake is _____ mg per day.

18. Dietary sources of calcium include which of the following? Select all that apply.

_____ Leafy green vegetables

_____ Cheese

_____ Seafood

_____ Legumes

_____ Sweet potatoes

_____ Canned fish with bones

_____ Egg yolks

19. The following medications have been ordered for Kathryn Doyle. Match each medication with its correct classification/usage. (*Hint:* Refer to the Drug Guide for assistance.)

	Medication	Classification
_____	Calcium citrate	a. Iron preparation; hematinic
_____	Ferrous sulfate	b. Stool softener
_____	Docusate sodium	c. Nonsteroidal antiinflammatory; antipyretic; nonnarcotic analgesic
_____	Ibuprofen	d. Antipyretic; nonnarcotic analgesic
_____	Oxycodone	e. Anitosteoporotic; antacid; phosphate adsorbent
_____	Acetaminophen	f. Schedule II narcotic analgesic; opiate derivative

20. What relationship does the nurse need to be aware of between the calcium citrate and the ferrous sulfate? How will this relationship affect the manner of administration?

21. Which of the following should be told to clients taking ferrous sulfate? Select all that apply.

_____ Stools will darken in color.

_____ Stools may appear clay-colored.

_____ Take the medication on an empty stomach to avoid nausea.

_____ Take the medication after meals or with food if GI discomforts occur.

_____ Do not take the medication with milk or eggs.

_____ This medication may reduce the effectiveness of some antibiotics.

Alterations in Nutrition: Gastrointestinal Dysfunction

Reading Assignment: Promoting Healthy Nutrition (Chapter 24)
Restoring Nutrition (Chapter 25)
Maintaining Fluid and Electrolyte Balance (Chapter 26)

Client: Piya Jordan, Medical-Surgical Floor, Room 403

Objectives:

1. Describe the functions and processes of the gastrointestinal (GI) system.
2. Discuss tests and tools used in the assessment of GI functioning and proper nutrition.
3. Understand the purpose and proper administration of parenteral feeding.
4. Describe appropriate nursing care of a client with dysfunctional GI system.

Exercise 1

 Clinical Preparation: Writing Activity

 30 minutes

  1. The four main functions of the GI system are _____,

  _____, _____, and _____.

2. Match each gastrointestinal structure below with its appropriate digestive function.

Gastrointestinal Structure	Digestive Function
_____ Mouth	a. No known function
_____ Colon	b. Closes when food is swallowed to prevent aspiration
_____ Epiglottis	
	c. Secretes bile for the emulsification of fat
_____ Esophagus	
	d. Mixes food with saliva
_____ Pancreatic duct	
	e. Finishes digestion of chyme and absorption across a smaller number of villi, especially at the distal end
_____ Ilium	
_____ Appendix	
	f. Reabsorbs water and electrolytes and prepares waste for excretion
_____ Liver	
_____ Pyloric sphincter	g. Transports food bolus from mouth to stomach
	h. Collects pancreatic enzymes and transports them to the duodenum
	i. Prevents backflow of alkaline intestinal contents into stomach

3. Indicate whether each of the following statements is true or false.

a. _____ Metabolism is the passage of the products of carbohydrates and proteins through the intestinal wall into the bloodstream for distribution throughout the body.

b. _____ Swallowing is an involuntary action controlled by the peripheral nervous system.

4. A phenomenon in which the body obtains glucose from protein in a process known as gluconeogenesis is referred to as _____.

5. A client has difficulty swallowing. When planning food options for the client, which of the following foods should be included? Select all that apply.

_____ Lukewarm foods

_____ Cold foods

_____ Mildly sweetened foods

_____ Pureed foods

_____ Moist pastas

6. Which of the following events can increase the body's nutritional needs? Select all that apply.

_____ Infection

_____ Fever

_____ Trauma

_____ Stress

_____ Rest

7. The nurse is performing a dietary assessment on a client. The most popular and easiest tool

to use is the _____.

8. _____ is the term used to refer to a condition caused by imbalanced, insufficient, or excessive diet or by impaired absorption or metabolism of nutrients.

9. The nurse is providing care for a client who is suspected of being malnourished. Which of the following diagnostic tests will best provide information to confirm these suspicions?
   a. Serum albumin
   b. Urinalysis
   c. Hematocrit
   d. Complete blood count

10. A client who is being evaluated for impaired nutritional status has a BUN test performed. The client's BUN is 4 mg/100 mL. Which of the following occurrences may be responsible for this imbalance?
   a. Excessive protein intake
   b. Zinc deficiency
   c. Protein wasting diseases
   d. Muscle wasting
   e. Low protein intake

 11. A student nurse notes that the vitamin and mineral content of the client's parenteral nutrition solution is less than the recommended daily amounts. What is the rationale for this discrepancy? (*Hint:* See page 607 in your textbook.)

12. When caring for a client who is receiving parenteral nutrition, the nurse is required to assess for signs and symptoms consistent with infection. Which of the following are symptoms associated with infection? Select all that apply.

_____ Hyperthermia

_____ Hypothermia

_____ Bradycardia

_____ Tachycardia

_____ Glucose intolerance

13. Radiography is the only definitive method to determine gastrostomy tube placement.
    a. True
    b. False

Exercise 2

CD-ROM Activity

45 minutes

- Sign in to work at Pacific View Regional Hospital on the Medical-Surgical Floor for Period of Care 2. (*Note:* If you are already in the virtual hospital from a previous exercise, click on **Leave the Floor** and then **Restart the Program** to get to the sign-in window.)
- From the Patient List, select Piya Jordan (Room 403).
- Click on **Get Report** and read the report.
- Click on **Go to Nurses' Station**.
- Click on **Chart** and then on **403** to view Piya Jordan's chart.
- Click on and review the **History and Physical** and **Nursing Admission** tabs.

1. Piya Jordan weight is _____ pounds (_____ kg). She is _____ inches tall.

2. Using the "at a glance" method, what is Piya Jordan's ideal weight? (*Hint:* See page 574 in your textbook.)

3. Piya Jordan reports a recent weight loss of _____ pounds.

4. List Piya Jordan's identified health care concerns.

➡ • Click on and review the **Laboratory Reports** tab.

5. Normal hematocrit levels are _____% to _____% for women.

6. Piya Jordan's hematocrit levels range from _____% to _____%.

7. Which of the following statements concerning the hematocrit are correct? Select all that apply.

_____ The hematocrit level indicates the body's protein level.

_____ Hematocrit is a measurement of the body's iron status.

_____ Hematocrit levels are the same for both men and women.

_____ Surgical intervention can alter the body's hematocrit levels.

_____ Dehydration is associated with a decrease in hematocrit.

8. Urine specific gravity is normally_____ to _____. Piya Jordan's urine specific

gravity is _____.

9. A reduced urine specific gravity is indicative of hypovolemia.
   a. True
   b. False

➡ • Click on and review the **Physician's Notes** and **Physician's Orders** tabs.

10. After _____ days without oral nutrition, enteral methods may be indicated.

11. What diet has been ordered for Piya Jordan?

12. What nutrition is being provided to Piya Jordan during this stage of her recovery?

13. Over the course of a 24-hour day, Piya Jordan will receive _____ mL of the D$_5$NS infusion.

14. Piya Jordan's prescribed intravenous fluids can best be described as:
    a. a Ringer's solution.
    b. a source of total parenteral nutrition.
    c. a hypotonic dextrose solution.
    d. an isotonic saline solution.
    e. a hypertonic dextrose solution.

15. The amount and type of the intravenous fluids being provided to Piya Jordan are adequate for preventing dehydration and for providing nutrition.
    a. True
    b. False

16. Which of the following statements best describes the intended action of Piya Jordan's ordered intravenous solution (D$_5$NS)?
    a. Mimics electrolyte concentration of blood
    b. Often used as a volume expander
    c. Provides energy and nutrients for cellular function and repair
    d. Expands extracellular fluid without changing osmolality

17. While caring for Piya Jordan, the nurse must frequently assess her IV site. The presence of complications can be identified by both manifestations at the site and observations of the client. Match each of the following complications with the appropriate signs and symptoms.

Complication	**Clinical Manifestation**
_____ Infiltration	a. Heat, pain, redness, and edema
_____ Phlebitis	b. Heat, pain, redness, edema, and possible fever and sepsis
_____ Infection	
_____ Air embolism	c. Fluid will not flow by gravity; site is edematous, blanched, painful, cold
_____ Allergic reaction	d. Rash, redness, itching
_____ Circulatory overload	e. Decreased blood pressure pressure; cyanosis and tachycardia
	f. Dyspnea, cough, cyanosis, jugular vein distention

18. A nasogastric (NG) tube may be used for which of the following reasons? Select all that apply.

    _____ Decompression—removal of secretions and gases from the GI tract.

    _____ Feeding—installation of liquid supplements or feedings into the stomach.

    _____ Compression—internal application of pressure by means of an inflated balloon to prevent internal GI hemorrhage.

    _____ Evacuation—reduction of intestinal stool contents

    _____ Lavage—irrigation of stomach; used in cases of active bleeding, poisoning, or gastric dilation

19. The nurse is planning to clean Piya Jordan's nostril where the NG tube is placed. Which of the following solutions is most appropriate for use?
    a. Use an alcohol-based solution
    b. Use mild soap and water
    c. Use hydrogen peroxide
    d. Use a water-soluble lubricant

20. When monitoring Piya Jordan's NG output, the nurse knows that which of the following findings may indicate fluid volume deficits? Select all that apply.

    _____ Hypotension

    _____ Pulse of more than 20 beats per minute above the baseline values

    _____ Hypertension

    _____ Urine production of less than 50 mL/hr for 2 or more consecutive hours

    _____ Confusion

21. Output totals of _____ mL or greater from the NG tube warrant notification of the physician.

LESSON 16 ——————————————————————

Bowel Elimination

———————————————————————————————

👓 **Reading Assignment:** Managing Bowel Elimination (Chapter 29)

Clients: Clarence Hughes, Medical-Surgical Floor, Room 404
Pablo Rodriguez, Medical-Surgical Floor, Room 405

Objectives:

1. Discuss problems of bowel elimination, including constipation, diarrhea, and bowel incontinence.
2. Explain the effect on bowel elimination of the client's diet and exercise, personal habits, cultural background, age and physiological and psychosocial factors.
3. Distinguish among the variety of nursing diagnoses for problems of bowel elimination.

Exercise 1

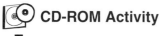 **CD-ROM Activity**

🕐 45 minutes

 1. Nursing responsibilities regarding bowel status include _____,

_____ of stool specimens, performing _____

_____, and _____ with physicians to meet the client's bowel elimination needs. (*Hint:* See page 718 of your textbook.)

2. Nurses should be aware that approximately _____ mL of water is excreted in waste materials by the body each day.

165

3. Match each of the following terms with its correct definition.

Term	Definition
_____ Feces	a. The process by which feces and flatus pass through the rectum and anal canal
_____ Peristalsis	b. Body waste discharged from the intestine
_____ Flatus	c. Collection of hardened feces in the rectum or sigmoid colon preventing passage of a normal stool
_____ Defecation	
_____ Valsalva maneuver	d. A condition in which feces are abnormally hard and dry
_____ Constipation	e. Rhythmic smooth muscle contractions that propel stool through the intestines
_____ Fecal impaction	f. Rapid movement of fecal matter through the intestine, resulting in diminished absorption of water, nutrients, and electrolytes
_____ Diarrhea	g. Swallowed air and gases produced through the digestive process
	h. Contraction of the abdominal muscles accompanied by an increased intrathoracic pressure against a closed glottis

4. The nurse is preparing to discuss the Valsalva maneuver with a client. Which of the following concepts are correct regarding this maneuver? Select all that apply.

_____ Valsalva maneuver is a concern for clients with a cardiac history.

_____ Valsalva maneuver may result during urination.

_____ Bearing down may illicit Valsalva maneuver.

_____ Intrathoracic pressure is increased during Valsalva maneuver.

_____ The glottis is open for a prolonged period during Valsalva maneuver.

5. The nurse is preparing to teach a client with a history of loose stools about how diet can help this condition. Increased consumption of which of the following food items would be beneficial for this client?
   a. Dairy products
   b. Eggs
   c. Rice
   d. Raw fruits
   e. Raw vegetables

6. A client who has had a recent ileostomy asks which foods may cause complications with defecation. Which of the following foods should the nurse advise the client to avoid? Select all that apply.

_____ Celery

_____ Corn

_____ Beer

_____ Chocolate

_____ Fresh fruits

_____ Nuts

7. What is the recommended daily amount of dietary fiber?
   a. 25 g
   b. 50 g
   c. 100 g
   d. 75 g

8. The bulk provided by dietary fiber assists _____ by increasing stimula-

   tion of the _____ reflex.

9. Foods high in fat content speed digestion and promote diarrhea.
   a. True
   b. False

10. A diet high in _____ is associated with a diminished defecation reflex.

11. When performing an assessment of bowel health in an older client, the nurse should consider which of the following factors? Select all that apply.

_____ Cavities or missing teeth may impair mastication.

_____ The amount of gastric juices in saliva increases with aging.

_____ Digestive enzymes in the stomach decrease with aging.

_____ Nerve impulses to the rectum are slowed with aging.

_____ The risk for cancer in the gastrointestinal system increases with aging.

12. When counseling a client concerning foods that may promote gas formation, a nurse should include which of the following food items in the discussion? Select all that apply.

_____ Radishes

_____ Onions

_____ Cheese

_____ Marshmallows

_____ Pasta

_____ Peanut butter

_____ Cola

13. List five categories of medications that may be prescribed to promote bowel regulation.

14. _____ are mixtures containing live bacteria, usually those species found in the gut, which can be used in the management of irritable bowel syndrome.

15. Which of the following is the best time to collect a specimen to assess for pinworms?
    a. In the evening before bedtime
    b. After the first bowel movement of the day
    c. Immediately upon arising
    d. After eating the morning meal
    e. After showering

16. Match each of the following fecal characteristics with its underlying cause.

Fecal Characteristic	Underlying Cause
_____ Brown stool	a. Bilary obstruction
_____ Light-colored stool	b. Normal function
_____ White stool	c. Malabsorption of fat
_____ Gray stool with observable mucus ingestion	d. Antacid ingestion
_____ Tarry or black stool	e. Intestinal bleeding

17. Which of the following food items may affect Hemoccult readings? Select all that apply.

_____ Chicken

_____ Steak

_____ Bread

_____ Orange juice

_____ Parsnips

_____ Watermelon

_____ Peaches

18. Match each of the following data clusters with its appropriate nursing diagnosis.

Data Cluster

_____ A 93-year-old male has begun to experience bowel incontinence during periods of confusion.

_____ A 65-year-old client has been experiencing diarrhea and an elevated temperature for the past 36 hours.

_____ A 54-year-old quadriplegic client has not had a bowel movement for the past 3 days.

_____ A client has been taking narcotic analgesics to manage a recent back injury.

Nursing Diagnosis

a. Constipation related to physical limitations

b. Diarrhea related to infectious processes

c. Bowel incontinence related to impaired cognition

d. Constipation related to medication therapy

19. A BRATY diet has been recommended for a client who has been experiencing gastroenteritis. Identify what each letter stands for in this acronym.

B:

R:

A:

T:

Y:

20. A cleansing enema is used for which of the following purposes? Select all that apply.

    _____ To clean the bowel in preparation for a diagnostic procedure

    _____ To aid in the establishment of regular bowel function

    _____ To lubricate a hardened fecal mass

    _____ For administration of medications

    _____ To destroy intestinal parasites

21. A cleansing enema should not be given more often than every _____ days.

22. Match each type of enema with its corresponding ingredient.

Enema	**Ingredient**
_____ Hypotonic	a. Tap water
_____ Hypertonic	b. Mineral oil
_____ Isotonic	c. Sodium phosphate
_____ Soap	d. Castile
_____ Oil	e. Normal saline

23. Stools can be liquid, unformed, soft, or hard. The consistency of the stool is a reflection of

    its _____ content.

24. Stools have a characteristically pungent order. To which of the following can the odor of the stool be attributed?

    _____ Bacteria

    _____ High water intake

    _____ Foods

    _____ Upper respiratory infection

    _____ Blood in the GI tract

Exercise 2

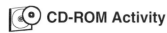 **CD-ROM Activity**

 60 minutes

- Sign in to work at Pacific View Regional Hospital on the Medical-Surgical Floor for Period of Care 1. (*Note:* If you are already in the virtual hospital from a previous exercise, click on **Leave the Floor** and then **Restart the Program** to get to the sign-in window.)
- From the Patient List, select Clarence Hughes (Room 404).
- Click on **Get Report** and read the report.
- Click on **Go to Nurses' Station** and then on **404**.
- Click on and review the **Clinical Alerts**.
- Click on **Patient Care** and then on **Nurse-Client Interactions**.
- Select and view the videos titled **0730: Assessment/Perception of Care** and **0735: Empathy**. (*Note:* Check the virtual clock to see whether enough time has elapsed. You can use the fast-forward feature to advance the time by 2-minute intervals if the videos are not yet available. Then click again on **Patient Care** and **Nurse-Client Interactions** to refresh the screen.)
- After the video, click on **Patient Care** and perform a complete systems assessment.

1. What are the two primary complaints being voiced by Clarence Hughes at this time?

- Click on **Chart** and then on **404**.
- Click on and review the **Nursing Admission** tab.

2. Normally, how often does Clarence Hughes have a bowel movement?

3. Review the characteristics of his last reported bowel movement. (*Hint:* See page 7 of the Nursing Admission.)

4. Are Clarence Hughes' typical bowel habits normal for a client of his age and gender?

5. Which of the following surgery-related events has the most bearing on Clarence Hughes' current state of constipation?
   a. Direct handling of the bowel during the operative procedure
   b. The onset of a paralytic ileus
   c. Postoperative edema at the site of the surgical intervention
   d. Administration of operative and postoperative medications

→ • Click on **Return to Room 404**.
   • Click on MAR and review the medications prescribed for Clarence Hughes.

6. Which of the medications prescribed for Clarence Hughes may promote constipation? Select all that apply. (*Hint:* If needed, click on the **Drug** icon for reference information.)

   _____ Docusate sodium

   _____ Celecoxib

   _____ Timolol maleate

   _____ Pilocarpine 1% ophthalmic solution

   _____ Enoxaparin

   _____ Promethazine hydrochloride

   _____ Magnesium hydroxide

   _____ Aluminum hydroxide with magnesium simethicone

   _____ Bisacodyl

   _____ Acetaminophen

   _____ Temazepam

   _____ Oxycodone with acetaminophen

7. In which position should Clarence Hughes be placed to best assess the abdomen?
   a. Prone
   b. Supine
   c. High Fowler's
   d. Semi-Fowler's

8. When visualizing Clarence Hughes' abdomen, what should the nurse be looking for?

9. The auditory characteristics of Clarence Hughes' bowel sounds may provide clues to conditions within the bowel.
   a. True
   b. False

10. During the abdominal assessment, the abdomen should be approached as divided into four

    _____.

11. The presence of a dull sound with percussion is indicative of:
    a. Air
    b. The onset of a paralytic ileus
    c. Feces
    d. Bladder distention

12. _____ are agents that stimulate defecation, and _____
    are strong laxatives that produce a watery stool.

13. Match each of the following laxative types with its correct description.

Laxative	Description
_____ Bulk-forming laxative	a. An osmotic agent that draws water into the intestine to increase bulk and lubricate feces
_____ Lubricant laxative	b. Synthetic or natural polysaccharides and cellulose derivative used to absorb water and increase stool volume, which will stimulate peristalsis
_____ Saline laxative	c. Works to increase peristalsis by stimulating sensory nerve endings of the colonic epithelium or by irritation of the GI mucosa
_____ Stimulant	d. Provides a coating of the outer fecal mass, which makes it slippery and inhibits fluid absorption

14. Match each of the following laxatives with its appropriate classification. (*Note:* You may use some classifications more than once.)

Laxative	Classification
_____ Bran	a. Stimulant
_____ Colace	b. Bulk-forming
_____ Magnesium hydroxide	c. Osmotic agent
_____ Bisacodyl	d. Lubricant laxative
_____ Dialose	
_____ Lactulose	

15. Which medications have been prescribed to manage Clarence Hughes' constipation?

- Prepare to administer Clarence Hughes' magnesium hydrochloride.
- Click on **Return to Room 404** and then on **Medication Room**.
- Click on **Unit Dosage** and then drawer **404**.
- Click on **Magnesium hydroxide** and then **Put Medication on Tray**. (*Hint:* You can review the MAR at any time to verify the physician's orders.)
- Click on **Close Drawer** and then on **View Medication Room**.
- Click on **Preparation** and then on **Prepare** next to the correct medication. Follow the Preparation Wizard's prompts.
- You can **Review Your Medications** and then **Return to Medication Room** when ready.
- Click on **404** to go to Clarence Hughes' room.
- Click on **Patient Care** and then on **Medication Administration**.
- Next to magnesium hydroxide, select **Administer** and follow the Administration Wizard's prompts.

16. The dosage of medication obtained was _____ mL.

17. When preparing the magnesium hydroxide, the nurse should measure the dose at the base of the meniscus. (*Hint:* See Chapter 21 in your textbook.)
    a. True
    b. False

18. The physician has also ordered a bisacodyl suppository. This medication will act as a

_____ to stimulate GI _____

_____.

19. Once the suppository is administered, how long should the client attempt to retain it?
   a. 5-10 minutes
   b. 20-30 minutes
   c. 1-2 hours
   d. Overnight

Exercise 3

 CD-ROM Activity

 45 minutes

- Sign in to work at Pacific View Regional Hospital on the Medical-Surgical Floor for Period of Care 2. (*Note:* If you are already in the virtual hospital from a previous exercise, click on **Leave the Floor** and then **Restart the Program** to get to the sign-in window.)
- From the Patient List, select Pablo Rodriguez (Room 405).
- Click on **Get Report** and read the report.
- Click on **Go to Nurses' Station** and then on **405**.
- Click and review **Clinical Alerts**.

1. In the change-of-shift report, what are Pablo Rodriguez's primary complaints?

 - Click on **Chart** and then on 405.
- Click on and review the **Nursing Admission** and **Physician's Notes** tabs.

2. What is Pablo Rodriguez's medical diagnosis?

3. Why is Pablo Rodriguez being admitted to the hospital?

4. Pablo Rodriguez's last bowel movement was _____.

5. Describe Pablo Rodriguez's last bowel movement.

➤ • Click on and review the **Nurse's Notes** tab.

6. According to the 1100 Nurse's Note, a mineral oil enema was administered to Pablo
    Rodriguez. How does this type of enema work?
    a. It lubricates the feces.
    b. It causes colon distention.
    c. It promotes peristalsis.
    d. It softens the fecal matter.

7. Which of the following positions is recommended when the client is being given an enema?
    a. Standing
    b. Client lying prone
    c. Client in right side-lying position
    d. Client in left side-lying position

8. The client should attempt to retain the mineral oil enema for _____ minutes.

9. Enemas should be given no more than every _____ days.

10. How often has the physician ordered the mineral oil enema?

11. A large-volume enema consists of how many mL of fluid?
    a. 250-500 mL
    b. 100-200 mL
    c. 500-1000 mL
    d. Greater than 1000 mL

➡ • Click on **Return to Room 405**.
  • Click on and review the **Initial Observations** and **Clinical Alerts**.
  • Click on **Patient Care** and perform a complete systems assessment.

12. Which of the following assessment findings are consistent with constipation?
    a. Characteristics of the bowel sounds
    b. Abdominal contour
    c. Skin temperature
    d. Vital signs

13. Which of the following factors is most responsible for Pablo Rodriguez's constipation?
    a. Dehydration
    b. Age
    c. Psychosocial considerations
    d. Immobility

➡ • Click on **MAR** and review Pablo Rodriguez's ordered medications.

14. Which of the ordered medications may contribute to Pablo Rodriguez's constipation? Select all that apply.

    _____ Morphine sulfate

    _____ Metoclopramide hydrochloride

    _____ Dexamethasone

    _____ Senna

    _____ Lactulose

    _____ Neutra-Phos

    _____ Ondansetron hydrochloride

15. The medications below have been ordered to manage Pablo Rodriguez's constipation. Match each the medications with its method of action.

Medication	Method of action
_____ Senna	a. Promotes increased peristalsis
_____ Lactulose	b. Stimulates the smooth muscle of the GI tract
_____ Neutra-Phos	c. Produces distention in the bowel

LESSON 17

Urinary Elimination

 Reading Assignment: Managing Urinary Elimination (Chapter 30)

Client: Piya Jordan, Medical-Surgical Floor, Room 403

Objectives:

1. Identify common problems of urinary elimination.
2. Discuss factors affecting urinary elimination.
3. Assess urinary function.
4. Implement basic nursing care for a client experiencing problems with urinary elimination.

Exercise 1

Clinical Preparation: Writing Activity

30 minutes

1. The waste products of urine include _UREA_, _Creatinine_, _uric acid_, and the products of hemoglobin breakdown.

2. The kidneys excrete or conserve sodium in response to _the bodys need_
blood levels of Na+.

179

3. Match each of the following terms with its correct definition.

Term	Definition
_d_ Micturition	a. Difficult or painful urination
_a_ Dysuria	b. Reoccurring involuntary urination that occurs during sleep
_c_ Oliguria	c. Diminished, scant amounts of urine
_e_ Anuria	d. The process of emptying the bladder
_f_ Polyuria	e. The absence of urine
_b_ Enuresis	f. The production of an excess of urine
_g_ Nocturia	g. Urination at nighttime

4. The color of normal urine may be ~~amber~~ pale straw colored, ~~dark amber~~, or ~~Bright yellow~~ clear.

5. Bright yellow urine may be associated with which of the following factors?
   a. Medication therapy
   b. Vitamin therapy
   c. The presence of bilirubin
   d. Reduced fluid intake

6. Urine darkens once it is outside of the body.
   a. True
   b. False

7. Which of the following may be associated with cloudy urine? Select all that apply.

   _____ Diabetes

   ✓ Bacteria

   ✓ Sperm

   _____ Vitamin therapy

   _____ Water intoxication

   _____ A diet high in vegetable intake

   ✓ Inflammation

8. Acidification of the urine can be achieved by which of the following interventions?

_____ Increasing the water intake

___✓___ Restricting dairy products

_____ Sodium bicarbonate

___✓___ Dietary modification

___✓___ Drinking cranberry juice

9. Women are more likely than men to experience urinary incontinence.
   ⓐ True
   b. False

10. Drugs associated with reduced control of urinary elimination include which of the following? Select all that apply.

___✓___ Sedatives

_____ Minerals

___✓___ Diuretics

___✓___ Immunosuppressants

_____ Vitamins

_____ Stool softeners

Exercise 2

 CD-ROM Activity

 45 minutes

- Sign in to work at Pacific View Regional Hospital on the Medical-Surgical Floor for Period of Care 1. (*Note:* If you are already in the virtual hospital from a previous exercise, click on **Leave the Floor** and then **Restart the Program** to get to the sign-in window.)
- From the Patient List, select Piya Jordan (Room 403).
- Click on **Get Report** and read the report.
- Click **Go to Nurses' Station** and then on **403**.
- Click on and review the **Clinical Alerts**.
- Click on **Patient Care** and perform a complete systems assessment.

1. Why has Piya Jordan been admitted to the hospital?

   Bowel obstruction

2. Is Piya Jordan's urine normal in appearance?

No, dark yellow-clear

3. Which of the following catheter types is being used by Piya Jordan?
   a. Texas catheter
   b. Straight catheter
   c. Condom catheter
   d. Foley catheter
   e. Irrigation catheter
   f. Suprapubic

4. Indicate whether each of the following statements is true or false.

   a. *True* Urinary catheterization is a high-risk factor for urinary tract infection.

   b. *True* A Foley catheter has a higher rate of infection than a suprapubic catheter.

   c. *False* Piya Jordan's catheter may be safely attached to the movable side rails of the bed.

5. Which of the following is the best location for the nurse to place the urinary collection bag?
   a. In the bed with the client
   b. On the client's chest
   c. Below the level of the client's bladder
   d. Above the level of the client's bladder

6. Bladder spasms may be a normal occurrence with an indwelling catheter. Which of the following interventions may be used to manage the condition? Select all that apply.

   ✓ Manipulate the catheter

   ____ Irrigate the catheter

   ____ Reduce fluid intake

   ✓ Increase fluid intake

   ____ Increase the size of the balloon that is holding the catheter in the bladder

   ____ Raise the catheter to shift the flow of urine back into the bladder

7. When providing catheter care for Piya Jordan, the nurse should use which of the following?
   a. Soap and water
   b. Hydrogen peroxide
   c. Neosporin
   d. Saline and water
   e. A solution with equal parts rubbing alcohol and water

8. What information concerning Piya Jordan's catheter should be documented in the progress notes?

patency, color of urine, amount of urine

Foley in place draining clear yellow urine in sufficient quantities

9. After the catheter is removed, Piya Jordan may experience urinary retention. Which of the following factors may be associated with this occurrence?
   a. The presence of a malignancy
   b. An elevated urine specific gravity
   c. Gender
   d. Medications used during the surgical procedure

10. After an indwelling catheter is removed, issues with residual urine volumes are most often permanent.
    a. True
    b. False

11. Piya Jordan's bladder should be palpated for the presence of *distension*

    _____. If present, this signals a possible obstruction in urine flow.

➤ • Click on **Chart** and then on **403**.
   • Click on and review the **Laboratory Reports**, **History and Physical**, and **Nursing Admission** tabs.

12. Which of the following factors have an impact on the urinary functioning of Piya Jordan? Select all that apply.

    _✓_ Aging

    ____ An increase in the number of functional nephrons in the kidneys

    _✓_ Reduced bladder capacity

    ____ Inability to urinate at night

    _✓_ Hormonal changes

13. Which of the following terms can be used to refer to Piya Jordan's urinary concerns prior to admission?
    a. Stress incontinence
    b. Functional incontinence
    c. Reflex urinary incontinence
    d. Psychological incontinence

14. Which of the following is most likely an underlying cause of the condition discussed in the previous question?
   a. Bladder outlet obstruction
   b. Voluntary muscle dysfunction
   c. Infection
   (d) Changes in pelvic floor muscles
   e. Neuromuscular limitations

15. __Uvinalysis__ is a physical, chemical, and microscopic examination of urine.

16. Normal urine specific gravity is __1.003__ to __1.030__.

17. Piya Jordan's urine specific gravity is __1.05__.

18. To what can Piya Jordan's urine specific gravity be attributed?

   dehydration

LESSON 18
_____

Respiratory Function

_____

👓 **Reading Assignment:** Supporting Respiratory Function (Chapter 34)

Client: Jacquline Catanazaro, Medical-Surgical Floor, Room 402

Objectives:

1. Discuss common lifestyle, environmental, developmental, and physiological factors affecting respiration.
2. Discuss common pathological conditions affecting respiration.
3. Assess the client at risk for responses to a respiratory problem.
4. Diagnose the client's respiratory needs that are amenable to nursing care.
5. Plan goal-directed interventions to prevent or correct the respiratory diagnoses.
6. Describe and practice key interventions for respiratory care, including positioning, suctioning, providing supplemental oxygen, and maintaining a patent (open) airway.

Exercise 1

 Clinical Preparation: Writing Activity

30 minutes

1. Match each of the following terms with its correct definition.

Term	Definition
_____ Ventilation	a. The measure of distention of the lungs
_____ Compliance	b. High carbon dioxide levels in the blood
_____ Elastic recoil	c. Volume of air remaining in the lungs after a maximum exhalation
_____ Airway resistance	
_____ Hypoxemia	d. The tendency of the lungs to return to a nonstretched state
_____ Hypercapnia	e. Deficient blood oxygen levels
_____ Tidal volume	f. The cycle of inspiration and expiration of air into and out of the lungs
_____ Residual volume	
_____ Vital capacity	g. Volume of air in lungs after maximal inhalation
_____ Total lung capacity	h. Volume of air forcefully exhaled after a maximum inhalation
_____ Forced breathing capacity (FVC)	i. Volume of air inhaled and exhaled with each normal respiration
	j. Opposition of airflow within air passages
	k. Volume of air remaining in the lungs at the end of normal expiration

2. The three important sets of accessory muscles are the _____,

   _____, and _____.

3. The mucous membranes of the upper airways function to _____,

   _____, and _____ the air.

4. Indicate whether each of the following statements is true or false.

   a. _____ You are scheduled to care for an 11-month-old client diagnosed with pneumonia. The client's age reduces the severity of this disease.

   b. _____ Fewer than half of all people who receive nicotine replacement are able to successfully quit smoking.

5. Match each of the following respiratory disorders with its appropriate description.

Respiratory Disorder

_____ Atelectasis

_____ Pleural effusion

_____ Hemothorax

_____ Pneumothorax

_____ Pneumoconiosis

_____ Pneumonia

_____ Asthma

_____ Emphysema

_____ Tuberculosis

Description

a. Inflammation of the lung with consolidation and exudation

b. Accumulation of fluid in the space between the visceral pleura and parietal pleura of the thorax

c. A collapsed or airless state of the lung or a portion of a lung

d. An infectious, inflammatory, reportable disease that is chronic in nature and commonly affects the lungs, although it may occur in almost any part of the body

e. An inflammatory response that constricts the bronchi and causes edema and increased production of sputum

f. Bleeding into the pleural space secondary to trauma to the chest

g. Pathological accumulation of air in tissues or organs

h. Air from the lung leaking into the pleural space or chest

i. A group of fibrotic lung diseases caused by prolonged inhalation of dust particles, usually from industrial dust; eventually develops a chronic obstructive component

6. You are preparing an educational program concerning respiratory health. Which of the following concepts is correct? Select all that apply.

_____ The most prominent risk factor for the development of respiratory disorders in adults is smoking.

_____ The amount of surfactant produced in the lungs increases with aging.

_____ Inactivity increases the risk for the development of respiratory-related complications.

_____ Dead insects have been investigated as an allergen in low-income housing.

_____ The lack of surfactant production in infants may result in hyaline membrane disease.

_____ The incidence of asthma is declining.

7. A nurse is providing postprocedural care for a client who has had a bronchoscopy. Which of the following positions would be the most therapeutic for the client?
   a. High Fowler's
   b. Semi-Fowler's
   c. Supine
   d. Prone

8. A client is being evaluated for tuberculosis. Which of the following diagnostic tests will provide the best clues related to this disorder?
   a. Complete blood count
   b. Chest radiograph
   c. Arterial blood gases
   d. Pulse oximetry

9. A bronchoscopy provides direct visualization of the _____,

   _____, and _____ using a flexible, fiberoptic scope.

10. _____ in the blood carries 97% of the oxygen, and the remaining 3% is

    dissolved in the _____.

11. A client is demonstrating hypoventilation. Which of the following PaCO2 readings can be expected for this client?
    a. Less than 31 mm Hg
    b. 32-40 mm Hg
    c. 41 mm Hg
    d. 47 mm Hg

12. Hypoventilation is defined as a respiratory rate of fewer than _____ breaths per minute.

13. When hypoventilation is being considered, why is the carbon dioxide level used instead of the oxygen level?

14. Which of the following factors may be associated with hypoventilation? Select all that apply.

_____ Exercise intolerance

_____ Immobility

_____ Pain

_____ Medications

_____ Muscle or nerve dysfunction

_____ Abdominal trauma

15. Identify the mechanisms used in chest physiotherapy. Select all that apply.

_____ Coughing

_____ Chest percussion

_____ Vibration

_____ Postural drainage

_____ Gravity

16. Gastrointestinal symptoms are of immediate concern in identifying hypoxemia.
    a. True
    b. False

17. Positioning a client on the _____ side may activate the cough reflex.

18. During the postoperative period, the client should be repositioned at least every _____ hours.

Exercise 2

 CD-ROM Activity

60 minutes

- Sign in to work at Pacific View Regional Hospital on the Medical-Surgical Floor for Period of Care 1. (*Note:* If you are already in the virtual hospital from a previous exercise, click on **Leave the Floor** and then **Restart the Program** to get to the sign-in window.)
- From the Patient List, select Jacquline Catanazaro (Room 402).
- Click on **Get Report** and read the report.
- Click on **Go to Nurses' Station**.
- Click on **Chart** and then on **402**.
- Click on and review the **Nursing Admission** and **History and Physical** tabs.

1. What are Jacquline Catanazaro's medical diagnoses?

2. Which of the following risk factors for the development of respiratory illness does Jacquline Catanazaro have? Select all that apply.

_____ Age

_____ History of travel

_____ Occupational exposures

_____ Smoking

_____ Family history

_____ Inactivity

→ • Click on **Return to Nurses' Station** and then on **402**.
   • Review the **Initial Observations**.
   • Click on and review the **Clinical Alerts**.
   • Click on **Take Vital Signs** and review the readings.

3. Identify Jacquline Catanazaro's current vital signs.

   Temperature:

   Heart rate:

   Respiratory rate:

   Blood pressure:

4. The normal respiratory rate for an adult is _____ to _____ per minute.

5. The pulse oximeter is a reading of the:
   a. level of the blood's hematocrit level.
   b. oxygen saturation of hemoglobin in the blood.
   c. body's level of $PaCO_2$.
   d. body's acid base balance.

6. Jacquline Catanazaro's pulse oximeter reading is _____%.

7. A saturation of _____% is the critical value for oxygenation to support life.

8. Which of the following may affect pulse oximeter readings?

_____   Hypertension

_____   Vasodilation

_____   Hypothermia

_____   Dark-colored nail polish

_____   Finger movement

→ • Click on **Patient Care** and complete a systems assessment.

9. Identify the abnormalities found during Jacquline Catanazaro's respiratory assessment.

10. If you were asked to describe the "crackles" heard in Jacquline Catanazaro's lung fields, what words would best be used?
    a. Continuous sonorous sounds
    b. High-pitched musical tones
    c. Low-pitched whistling sounds
    d. Bubbling sounds

11. Another term that may used interchangeably with "crackles" is:
    a. rhonchi.
    b. wheezes.
    c. friction rub.
    d. alveolar popping.

12. The respiratory assessment reflects the presence of wheezes. Which of the following best describes the underlying causes of the wheezing sound?
    a. Pulmonary hypoventilation
    b. Mucus in the bronchioles
    c. Inflammation of the pleura
    d. Bronchoconstriction
    e. Fluid overload

13. Jacquline Catanazaro is demonstrating an increased respiratory rate. Which of the following can result in an increase in respiratory rate? Select all that apply.

_____ Exercise

_____ Fever

_____ Alkalosis

_____ Hypoxemia

_____ Hypercapnia

14. During the respiratory crisis being experienced by Jacquline Catanazaro, what is the priority nursing diagnosis?
    a. Activity intolerance
    b. Anxiety
    c. Impaired gas exchange
    d. Ineffective health maintenance

15. Jacquline Catanazaro's skin is noted as being moist and clammy. What significance does this have in relation to her respiratory status? (*Hint:* See page 901 in your textbook.)

16. When an asthmatic condition is suspected, which of the following diagnostic tests should be ordered to confirm a diagnosis? Select all that apply.

_____ Complete blood count

_____ Serum electrolyte levels

_____ Arterial blood gas levels

_____ Pulmonary function tests

_____ Sputum cultures

→ • In response to Jacquline Catanazaro's respiratory distress, the physician is notified at 0730.
  • Click on **Chart** and then on **402**.
  • Click on the **Physician's Orders** tab and review the orders received at 0730 and 0800.

17. Match each of the stat medications ordered with its correct classification.

Medication	Classification
_____ Albuterol	a. Corticosteroid
_____ Beclomethasone	b. Bronchodilator
_____ Methylprednisolone sodium succinate	c. Corticosteroid, antiinflammatory

18. At 0730 the physician ordered albuterol. How long can Jacquline Catanazaro expect to wait for the medication to begin to work?

19. Which of the following instructions should the nurse give to Jacquline Catanazaro about administering albuterol? Select all that apply.

_____ Shake container before use

_____ Hold container at a 45-degree angle during administration

_____ Exhale fully while depressing top of canister

_____ Wait 2 minutes before inhaling second dose

_____ Avoid water intake immediately after administration

20. Arterial blood gas levels are measured to determine the partial pressures of oxygen and carbon dioxide as an indicator of respiratory function.
    a. True
    b. False

21. What clinical manifestations would indicate improvement in Jacquline Catanazaro's condition?

- Click on **Return to Room 402**.
- Click on **MAR** and then on **402**.
- Review the medications ordered for this period of care.

22. Amoxicillin 500 mg is ordered for 0800. What is the rationale for the administration of this medication?
    a. To manage infection
    b. To increase lung expansion
    c. To reduce the heart rate
    d. To increase cardiac output

- Click on **Return to Room 402**.
- Click on **Medication Room**.
- Click on **MAR** and then on **402** to determine the medications that Jacquline Catanazaro is ordered to receive. (*Note:* Remember to look at the client name on the MAR to make sure you have the correct record—you must click on the correct room number within the MAR.)
- Click on **Return to Medication Room** after reviewing the correct MAR.
- Click on **Unit Dosage** and then on drawer **402**.
- Choose **Amoxicillin** and then **Put Medication on Tray**.
- Click on **Close Drawer** and then on **View Medication Room**.
- Click on **Preparation**; next to amoxicillin, click **Prepare**.
- Follow the Preparation Wizard's prompts to prepare this medication.
- You can **Review Your Medications** and then **Return to Medication Room** when ready. Once you are back in the Medication Room, go directly to Jacquline Catanazaro's room to administer this medication by clicking on **402** at the bottom of the screen.
- After you have collected the appropriate assessment data and are ready for administration, click **Patient Care** and then **Medication Administration**. Verify that the correct client and medication (s) appear on the left-hand window.
- Click the down arrow next to **Select**, and from the drop-down menu, choose **Administer** and complete the Administration Wizard's prompts by providing any information requested. When the Wizard stops asking for information, click **Administer to Patient**. Specify **Yes** when asked whether this administration should be recorded in the MAR. Finally, click **Finish**.
- Click on **Leave the Floor** and then **Look at Your Preceptor's Evaluation**. Choose **Medication Scorecard** and review you results.

LESSON **19**

Managing Pain

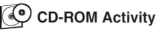 **Reading Assignment:** Managing Pain (Chapter 37)

Clients: Harry George, Medical-Surgical Floor, Room 401
Pablo Rodriguez, Medical-Surgical Floor, Room 405

Objectives:

1. Describe the physiological, cultural, lifestyle, and life span factors that affect the pain experience.
2. Assess the client experiencing or at risk for experiencing pain.
3. Assess the client's responses to the experience of pain.
3. Plan goal-directed interventions to prevent or correct the diagnosis of pain.
4. Describe and practice key nonpharmacological and pharmacological interventions for pain management.
5. Evaluate outcomes that indicate progress in providing effective pain management.

Exercise 1

CD-ROM Activity

 45 minutes

1. _____ is the process of transmitting a pain signal from a site of tissue damage to areas of the brain where perception occurs.

2. _____ are a group of internally secreted, opiate-like substances released in response to a signal from the cerebral cortex.

3. Match each of the following terms with its correct definition.

Key term	Definition
_____ Paresthesia	a. An unpleasant, abnormal sensation
_____ Dysesthesia	b. Diminished pain in response to a normally painful stimulus
_____ Allodynia	
_____ Hypoalgesia	c. Pain experienced at a site distant from the injured tissue
_____ Hyperalgesia	d. An abnormal sensation
_____ Somatic pain	e. Pain in response to a stimulus that does not normally provoke pain
_____ Visceral pain	
_____ Referred pain	f. Well localized pain, usually from bone or spinal metastases or from injury to cutaneous or deep tissues
	g. Painful syndrome characterized by an abnormally painful reaction to a stimulus, especially a repetitive stimulus, as well as an increased threshold
	h. Poorly localized pain

4. While caring for a client, you note the presence of agitation, insomnia, diarrhea, and sweating when requests for "strong" analgesics is refused by the physician. Which of the following should be suspected?
   a. The client has developed a tolerance to all analgesics.
   b. The client has developed psychological dependence.
   c. The client is an alcoholic and needs a drink.
   d. The client has developed physiological dependence.

5. Which of the following clients is most likely to benefit from a psychological assessment regarding pain?
   a. A 4-year-old client waiting to undergo an appendectomy
   b. A 32-year-old client recovering from a sprained ankle
   c. A 65-year-old client who has chronic pain associated with osteoporosis
   d. An 85-year-old male client who is planning to undergo a total hip replacement

6. A _____ is anything a person says or does that implies the presence of pain.

7. Match each of the following characteristics with the type of pain it is most likely to be associated with. (*Hint:* See page 1006 in your textbook.)

Characteristic	Type of Pain
_____ Usually responds to commonly prescribed medical and nursing interventions	a. Acute pain
_____ May not be associated with an identified injury or event	b. Chronic pain
_____ Consists of discomfort lasting 4 months	
_____ Includes evidence of tissue damage	
_____ May not be reported	

8. Indicate whether each of the following statements is true or false.

a. _____ Gender can affect an individual's pain threshold and tolerance.

b. _____ Pain in men is more likely to be undertreated.

c. _____ Pain is a normal occurrence of aging.

9. When the nurse if providing care for a Mexican-American client, which of the following traditional behaviors might be anticipated? Select all that apply.

_____ Attempts to maintain direct eye contact during all care interactions

_____ Remains silent when in agreement with the plan of care

_____ Keeps personal, sensitive issues private within the family

_____ Believes strongly that anxiety can hamper health status

_____ Believes strongly that self-care may promote a speedy recovery

10. If a client who has undergone surgery questions the use of narcotic analgesics and is concerned about becoming "addicted," which of the following responses by the nurse is most appropriate?
    a. "You should avoid the use of narcotics after the first postoperative day to reduce the incidence of addiction."
    b. "Addiction is an unfortunate but common event during the postoperative period."
    c. "Taking the ordered pain medicine every 6 hours will reduce the incidence of becoming addicted."
    d. "Addiction is not a common occurrence associated with postoperative pain management."
    e. "You should speak with your doctor about this concern."
    f. "Do you have a history of alcohol and drug dependency?"

11. Discuss the influence of culture on a client's beliefs about and experience of pain.

12. Which of the following clinical manifestations will the nurse most likely note for a client who is experiencing acute pain?
    a. Chilling, elevated heart rate, elevated blood pressure
    b. Elevated heart rate, elevated blood pressure, sweating
    c. Sweating, elevated temperature, elevated blood pressure, reduced heart rate
    d. Chilling, elevated blood pressure, reduced temperature, reduced heart rate

13. A nurse is assigned to provide care to a client who had surgery on the previous day. A pain assessment should be completed every _____ to _____ hours.

14. When providing care for a toddler, the nurse should consider which of the following behavioral manifestations as age-appropriate signs of pain? Select all that apply.

    _____ Vigorous body movements

    _____ Aggression

    _____ Crying

    _____ Screaming

    _____ Physically striking out

    _____ Verbally striking out

15. _____ refers to the dosages of different drugs that provide the same amount of pain relief.

16. A nurse is preparing to provide an in-service on the use of alternative treatments for pain. Which of the following concepts is correct and may be included in the presentation? Select all that apply.

    _____ Chiropractic treatments may increase client depression.

    _____ Massage therapy may lessen anxiety and depression.

    _____ Music therapy has no untoward side effects.

    _____ Unwillingness to be touched may hinder the success of massage therapy.

    _____ Music therapy is an expensive alternative for pain management.

17. Which of the following are associated with undertreatment of pain by health care providers? Select all that apply.

_____ Concerns about the cost of medications prescribed

_____ Inadequate information about the drugs ordered

_____ Anxiety about potential client injuries suffered while being medicated

_____ Laziness of the health care provider

_____ Concerns about fostering addiction

Exercise 2

CD-ROM Activity

45 minutes

- Sign in to work at Pacific View Regional Hospital on the Medical-Surgical floor for Period of Care 2. (*Note:* If you are already in the virtual hospital from a previous exercise, click on **Leave the Floor** and then **Restart the Program** to get to the sign-in window.)
- From the Patient List, select Harry George (Room 401).
- Click on **Get Report** and read the report.
- Click on **Go to Nurses' Station** and then on 401.
- Click on and review the **Clinical Alerts**.

1. Harry George is reporting a pain level of _____ on a 10-point scale.

2. The type of scale being used to assess Harry George's pain is known as a:
   a. visual analogue scale.
   b. numerical rating scale.
   c. verbal descriptor scale.
   d. linear pain continuum scale.

3. When selecting the type of pain scale to use, the nurse must consider the client's

   _____ of _____, _____, and

   _____.

- Click **Chart** and then on **401**.
- Click on and review the **Nursing Admission**, **History and Physical**, and **Physician's Notes** tabs.

4. What are Harry George's medical diagnoses?

5. What behavioral cues alluding to the presence of pain are being manifested by Harry George?

 • Click on **Return to Room 401**.
  • Click on **Patient Care** and then on **Physical Assessment** to complete a head-to-toe physical assessment of Harry George.

6. Based on the data collected from the physical assessment, which of the following types of pain is Harry George most likely experiencing?
   a. Somatic pain
   b. Visceral pain
   c. Referred pain
   d. Hypoanalgesic response
   e. Allodynia

 • Click on **EPR** and then on **Login**.
  • Select **401** as the patient and **Vital Signs** as the category.
  • Review the vital signs reported in the previous shifts.

7. Which of the following statements best explains the lack of notable changes in vital signs despite Harry George's complaints of severe pain? (*Hint:* See page 1008 in your textbook.)
   a. He is not experiencing the level of pain being reported.
   b. The alcohol detoxification process has caused him to complain excessively.
   c. There is no explanation for this phenomena.
   d. The sympathetic nervous system responses have abated, and the vital signs are now at his baseline.
   e. The parasympathetic nervous system responses have stalled, and the vital signs are not at the baseline.

8. Are Harry George's complaints of pain considered acute or chronic?

 • Click on **Exit EPR**.
  • Click on **MAR** and then on tab **401**.
  • Review Harry George's ordered medications.

9. According to the nurse's entry on the MAR, Harry George may be remedicated for

complaints of pain at _____.

10. When the nurse is planning care for Harry George, how long after the administration of hydromorphone hydrochloride should interventions be performed to ensure maximum effectiveness of the drug? (*Hint:* Refer to the Drug Guide as necessary.)
    a. 15 minutes
    b. 15-30 minutes
    c. 30-60 minutes
    d. 2 hours
    e. 3 hours

11. If the route of administration for the hydromorphone hydrochloride is changed to PO, what dosage can be anticipated if the level of pain requiring management remains the same?
    a. 2 mg
    b. 7.5 mg
    c. 4 mg
    d. No calculation available

12. Which of the following nursing diagnoses is most appropriate and has the highest priority for Harry George at this time?
    a. Activity intolerance
    b. Ineffective role performance
    c. Ineffective coping
    d. Hopelessness
    e. Disturbed body image
    f. Acute pain

Exercise 3

CD-ROM Activity

60 minutes

- Sign in to work at Pacific View Regional Hospital on the Medical-Surgical floor for Period of Care 2. (*Note:* If you are already in the virtual hospital from a previous exercise, click on **Leave the Floor** and then **Restart the Program** to get to the sign-in window.)
- From the Patient List, select Pablo Rodriguez (Room 405).
- Click on **Get Report** and read the report.
- Click on **Go to Nurses' Station** and then on **405**.
- Click on and review **Clinical Alerts**.

1. Presently, Pablo Rodriguez is reporting a pain level of _____ on a 10-point scale.

2. The pain associated with a diagnosis of cancer may be the result of

_____, _____,

and _____. (*Hint:* See page 1023 in your textbook.)

➥ • Click on **Chart** and then on **405**.
  • Click on and review the **Nursing Admission**, **Nurse's Notes**, **History and Physical**, and **Physician's Notes** tabs.

3. What are Pablo Rodriguez's medical diagnoses?

4. To treat/manage the cancer, Pablo Rodriguez has undergone chemotherapy and radiation therapy. Which of the following describes the manner in which these therapies are used to manage cancer. Select all that apply.

_____ Shrink the tumor

_____ Debulk the cancerous growths

_____ Reduce spinal cord compression

_____ Reduce pain from tumor metastases to the bone

_____ Alleviate painful nerve compression related to tumor infiltration

_____ Stabilize bony structures

➥ • Click on **Return to Room 405**.
  • Click on **Patient Care** and then on **Physical Assessment** to complete a head-to-toe physical assessment of Pablo Rodriguez.

5. Based on the assessment, which of the following are sources of discomfort for Pablo Rodriguez? Select all that apply.

_____ Condition of the oral cavity

_____ Constipation

_____ Ability to urinate

_____ Breathing

_____ Subcutaneous nodules

_____ Lymph nodes in the neck

→ • Click on **EPR** and then on **Login**.
  • Select **405** as the patient and **Vital Signs** as the category.
  • Review the information concerning Pablo Rodriguez's pain during this hospitalization.

6. During this hospitalization, the range of reported pain levels for Pablo Rodriguez has been

   between _____ and _____.

7. Which of the following characteristics are used to describe Pablo Rodriguez pain on Wednesday? Select all that apply.

   _____ Aching

   _____ Burning

   _____ Chronic

   _____ Dull

   _____ Electric

   _____ Intermittent

   _____ Internal

   _____ Sharp

   _____ Shooting

→ • Click **MAR** and then on tab **405**.
  • Review Pablo Rodriguez's ordered medications.

8. Match each of Pablo Rodriguez's ordered medications with its correct classification.

Medication	Classification
_____ Morphine sulfate	a. Antiemetic, blocks serotonin
_____ Metoclopramide hydrochloride	b. Ammonia detoxicant
_____ Mineral oil	c. Schedule II narcotic analgesic
_____ Zolpidem tartrate	d. Stool softener
_____ Dexamethasone	e. Schedule IV hypnotic
_____ Senna	f. Antiemetic, reduces esophageal reflux
_____ Lactulose	g. Laxative
_____ Ondansetron hydrochloride	h. Corticosteroid

9. The rationale for ordering two analgesics to manage Pablo Rodriguez's pain is that:
   a. providing the IV push medication will reduce his dependence on the PCA pump.
   b. having multiple analgesic orders will allow the client to choose which is preferred.
   c. this is a standard order.
   d. having the two medications provides a means to manage breakthrough pain.

10. Opioids have been ordered to manage Pablo Rodriguez's pain. Which of the following best describes the manner in which these medications work? (*Hint:* See page 1003 in your textbook.)
    a. Interfere with the relay of the pain signal across the synapse
    b. Inhibit prostaglandin synthesis
    c. Reduce serotonin availability to reduce pain occurrence
    d. Prevent and block the generation of the pain signals sent

11. In the list below, identify the potential side effects associated with opioid use. Select all that apply.

    _____ Diarrhea

    _____ Constipation

    _____ Drowsiness

    _____ Nausea

    _____ Hypertension

    _____ Bradycardia

    _____ Diaphoresis

12. Identify several nonpharmacologic interventions that can be used to manage Pablo Rodriguez's pain.

13. The MAR reports that Pablo Rodriguez has a continuous PCA pump with morphine sulfate PCA 1 mg/mL, 0.5 mg every 10 min/12 mg in 4-hour lockout. What is the maximum amount of morphine that may be delivered by the PCA pump in a 4-hour period?
    a. 10 mg
    b. 12 mg
    c. 6 mg
    d. 24 mg

14. Indicate whether each of the following statements is true or false.

   a. _____ Meperidine (Demerol) will likely be a suitable alternative for the manage-
      ment of Pablo Rodriguez's pain.

   b. _____ Dosages of morphine sulfate should be held if the client's respirations are
      less than 14 per minute.

➤ • Click on **Return to Room 405**.
   • Click on **Medication Room**.
   • Click on the **Automated System** and then on **Login**.
   • Click on **Review MAR** and then on tab **405**. Review the medication orders.
   • Click on **Return to Medication Room**.
   • Select **Pablo Rodriguez**, **405** and then **Automated System Drawer (G-O)**.
   • Click on **Open Drawer**.

15. The available strengths of the morphine sulfate that may be used for the IV push infusion

   are _____ and _____.

➤ • Select the appropriate strength of morphine sulfate.
   • Click on **Put Medication on Tray** and then **Close Drawer**.
   • Click on **View Medication Room**.
   • Click **Preparation** and then **Prepare**.
   • Follow the prompts of the Preparation Wizard to prepare the morphine sulfate.

16. How much medication will be drawn into the syringe?

17. The prepared dosage of morphine sulfate should be diluted with NS prior to administration.
   a. True
   b. False

18. The rapid administration of morphine sulfate IV push may be associated with which of the
   following complications? Select all that apply.

   _____ Minor anaphylactic reaction

   _____ Paresthesia at injection site

   _____ Severe anaphylactic reaction

   _____ Tachycardia

   _____ Apnea

   _____ Cardiac arrest

   _____ Circulatory collapse

19. After administration of IV push morphine sulfate, Pablo Rodriguez's vital signs should be

   assessed in _____ to _____ minutes.

- Click on **Return to Medication Room** and then on **405**.
- Click on **Patient Care** and then on **Medication Administration**.
- From the drop-down menu next to morphine sulfate, choose **Administer**.
- Follow the prompts of the Administration Wizard to administer the dose of morphine sulfate.
- Once you have finished, click on **Leave the Floor** and then on **Look at Your Preceptor's Evaluation** to review your medication administration.

LESSON **20** —————————————————————

Managing Loss

—————————————————————

👓 **Reading Assignment:** Managing Loss (Chapter 45)

Client: Goro Oishi, Skilled Nursing Floor, Room 505

Objectives:

1. Define the concepts of loss, grief, mourning/bereavement, death, and thanatology.
2. Compare and contrast the various types of loss and grieving.
3. Identify a variety of factors that affect the grief response.
4. Describe the assessment of a client or family member who is experiencing grief.
5. Describe the focused assessment of a dying client.
6. Plan nursing interventions used in caring for the dying client.

Exercise 1

 CD-ROM Activity

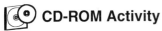 30 minutes

1. Match each of the following key terms with its correct definition.

Key term	Definition
_____ Palliative care	a. The philosophical concept of providing supportive care to the dying client
_____ Hospice care	
_____ Bereavement	b. Encompasses grief and mourning and denotes emotions and behaviors of one who experiences a loss
_____ Mourning	c. The study of death and death-related topics
_____ Thanatology	d. The active management of clients whose disease is not responsive to curative treatment
	e. The social and cultural acts and expressions used to convey thoughts and feelings of sorrow

2. _____ is the effort by a grieving person to acknowledge the physical and psychological pain associated with bereavement.

3. A _____ is an unexpected, involuntary resurgence of acute grief-related emotions and behaviors triggered by routine events.

4. Palliative care is designed to manage the last month of life.
   a. True
   b. False

5. Arrange the Elisabeth Kübler-Ross stages of death and dying in order of occurrence.

Stage	Order of Occurrence
_____ Acceptance	a. Stage 1
_____ Denial	b. Stage 2
_____ Bargaining	c. Stage 3
_____ Depression	d. Stage 4
_____ Anger	e. Stage 5

6. A client with terminal cancer announces to you that he promises to begin attending church regularly in hopes of a cure. Based on your knowledge, in which of the following Kübler-Ross stages of death and dying is this client?
a. Acceptance
b. Denial
c. Bargaining
d. Depression
e. Anger

7. The nurse is caring for a client who has been pronounced "brain dead" after an automobile accident. The client's wife begins to demonstrate somatic responses. Which of the following manifestations can be anticipated? Select all that apply.

_____ Muscle weakness

_____ Hypersensitivity to noise

_____ Dry mouth

_____ Tachycardia

_____ Bradycardia

_____ Chest tightness

_____ Dyspnea

8. Identify factors that may lessen the grief experienced by survivors.

9. While caring for a child who is terminally ill and nearing death, you overhear his mother arranging for him to enroll in school. The mother is demonstrating which of the following responses?
a. Selective attention
b. Deception
c. True denial
d. Anger
e. Compartmentalization

10. Identify risk factors associated with complicated grief. Select all that apply.

_____ Dependent relationships

_____ A lengthy, terminal illness

_____ History of alcohol abuse

_____ Current history of substance abuse

_____ Cumulative grief over multiple unresolved losses

11. When working with the family of a client who is nearing death, which of the following statements will facilitate the interaction? Select all that apply.

_____ "You are being strong."

_____ "I know how you feel."

_____ "I will keep you in my thoughts."

_____ "Time will make it easier."

_____ "You must get on with your life."

12. The wife of a man who died after a lingering illness reports that she has sold their home and plans to relocate in an effort to move forward. Which of the following tasks associated with grieving is the woman working through?
a. Recognition
b. Redirection
c. Reflection
d. Retribution

Exercise 2

 CD-ROM Activity

 60 minutes

• Sign in to work at Pacific View Regional Hospital on the Skilled Nursing floor for Period of Care 1. (*Note:* If you are already in the virtual hospital from a previous exercise, click on **Leave the Floor** and then **Restart the Program** to get to the sign-in window.)
• From the Patient List, select Goro Oishi (Room 505).
• Click on **Get Report** and read the report.
• Click on **Go to Nurses' Station**.
• Click on **Chart** and then on **505**.
• Click on and review the **History and Physical** tab.

1. Why was Goro Oishi admitted to the hospital? What is his current status?

2. What plans for care are identified in Goro Oishi's History and Physical?

3. Goro Oishi has been admitted for hospice care. Which of the following describe the components or features of a hospice care program? Select all that apply.

_____   A facility for treatment of terminal illnesses

_____   Treatment philosophy focused on symptom control

_____   Interdisciplinary care team approach

_____   Approach in which care providers set goals made to meet the family's desires

_____   Coordination of home care services

→ • Click on the **Physician's Notes** tab and read the progress notes.
  • Click on and review the **Consents** tab.

4. Because of Goro Oishi's incapacitation, who is controlling his medical care? Why is this person able to direct his care?

5. Which of the following statements regarding the roles of those in charge of Goro Oishi's health care is correct?
   a. Mrs. Oishi will have the authority to handle her husband's financial affairs.
   b. Mrs. Oishi will be required to consult with the entire family to obtain an consensus when making critical decisions.
   c. The physician will be required to make the final determination regarding the health care decisions.
   d. The Oishi family attorney will be required to go to court to make Mrs. Oishi her husband's health care guardian.
   e. Mrs. Oishi can make all of the health care decisions in the event that her husband is unable to make decisions for himself.

6. In the event Mrs. Oishi is unable or unwilling to make health care decisions for her husband, who will given the authority to do so?
   a. The physician will be in charge of making health care decisions.
   b. The hospital attorney will be in charge of making health care decisions.
   c. Goro Oishi's son will be in charge of making health care decisions.
   d. Goro Oishi will become a ward of the state.
   e. Goro Oishi's attorney will be in charge of making health care decisions.

7. If Goro Oishi's son does not agree with Mrs. Oishi, her wishes will be deemed invalid.
   a. True
   b. False

8. Ideally, who should be given copies of an advance directive prior to its being implemented? Select all that apply.

   _____ Members of the immediate family

   _____ A judge

   _____ The primary care physician

   _____ The nurses providing care

9. List the specific powers given to Mrs. Oishi by the advance directive.

➤ • Click on and review the **Nurse's Notes** tab.

10. The Nurse's Notes indicate the family is considering options regarding nutrition and IV therapy. If IV therapy and hydration is withheld, will Goro Oishi experience increased discomfort at the end of his life?

 • Click on **Return to Nurses' Station** and then on **505**.
• Review the **Initial Observations**.
• Click on **Take Vital Signs**.
• Click on **Patient Care** and then on **Physical Assessment** to complete a systems assessment.

11. Which of the following physical signs of imminent death are being exhibited by Goro Oishi? Select all that apply.

_____ Altered vital signs

_____ Decreased peripheral circulation

_____ Cyanotic and mottled extremities

_____ Cool, cold, or clammy extremities

_____ Fever

_____ Diminished skin turgor

_____ Edema

_____ Decreased urine output

12. The neurologic assessment and clinical report note Goro Oishi's Glasgow Coma Scale score. Which of the following are included in this assessment tool? Select all that apply. (*Hint:* Refer to a medical dictionary as needed.)

_____ Spontaneous eye opening

_____ Ability to demonstrate coherent speech patterns

_____ Orientation to person, place, and time

_____ Verbal responses

_____ Presence of spontaneous movement

13. Goro Oishi demonstrates decerebrate posturing. What does this mean? (*Hint:* Refer to a medical dictionary as needed.)
   a. All four extremities demonstrate rigid extension.
   b. The arms, wrists, and fingers demonstrate abnormal flexion.
   c. There is no response by the extremities to painful stimuli.
   d. The client is brain-dead.

 14. The assessment of Goro Oishi's pupil response indicates that the pupils are unequal and sluggish. Which cranial nerve is responsible for this manifestation? (*Hint:* Refer to Chapter 8 in your textbook, as necessary.)
   a. Cranial Nerve I: Olfactory
   b. Cranial Nerve II: Optic
   c. Cranial Nerve III: Oculomotor
   d. Cranial Nerve IV: Trochlear
   e. Cranial Nerve V: Trigeminal

 • Click on **Patient Care** and then on **Nurse-Client Interactions**.
   • Select and view the following videos:
      0730: Assessment—Patient
      0735: Assessment—Family
      0745: Intervention—Clarification
      0750: Family Conflict—Plan of Care
      0755: Death: The Right to Decide
      (*Note:* Check the virtual clock to see whether enough time has elapsed. You can use the fast-forward feature to advance the time by 2-minute intervals if the videos are not yet available. Then click again on **Patient Care** and **Nurse-Client Interactions** to refresh the screen.)

15. During the Nurse-Client Interaction at 0730, the nurse mentions the instillation of drops into Goro Oishi's eyes. What is the purpose of this intervention?

16. During the Nurse-Client Interaction at 0750, Kioshi Oishi is demonstrating which of the following stages associated with the grieving process?
   a. Recognition
   b. Retribution
   c. Reflection
   d. Reorganization

17. Goro Oishi's sons are demonstrating complicated grieving.
   a. True
   b. False

18. According to your textbook, there are five phases of communication with dying loved ones. Rank the phases in order of their occurrence.

Phases of Communication	**Order of Occurrence**
_____ Goodbye	a. Phase 1
_____ Forgive me	b. Phase 2
_____ I love you	c. Phase 3
_____ Thank you	d. Phase 4
_____ I forgive you	e. Phase 5

19. Identify one goal and outcome for the Oishi family during the dying process.

Surgery and Wound Care

👓 **Reading Assignment:** Promoting Wound Healing (Chapter 27)
The Surgical Client (Chapter 50)

Client: Piya Jordan, Medical-Surgical Floor, Room 403

Objectives:

1. Describe skin disruptions, wound healing, and problems of wound healing.
2. Explain the effects of lifestyle, age, and illness on skin integrity and wound healing.
3. Assess the client who is at risk for or has an impairment of skin integrity.
4. Identify factors that may affect the surgical outcome of a client.
5. Differentiate among general, regional, and local anesthesia.
6. Explain the nursing management of a client who has had surgery.

Exercise 1

CD-ROM Activity

45 minutes

1. Identify four functions of the dermis.

   1) gives structure + flexibility to the skin
   2) supplies nutrients
   3) removes wastes
   4) senses pain, touch, pressure, + temp

2. A ___lesion___ is a disruption of normal anatomical structure and function resulting from bodily injury or a pathological process.

3. Match each of the following types of wound drainage with its correct characteristics.

Drainage type

_b_ Serous

_d_ Sanguineous

_a_ Serosanguineous

_c_ Purulent

Characteristic

a. Pink, watery drainage consisting of plasma and red blood cells

b. Clear, watery plasma drainage

c. A protein-rich drainage that is the result of the liquefaction of necrotic tissue

d. Red drainage

4. When assigned to care for a surgical client with a history of diabetes, the nurse knows that which of the following events associated with the condition may increase the risk for development of complications? Select all that apply.

_✓_ Impaired tissue perfusion

_____ Increased red blood cell count

_✓_ Inhibition of leukocyte activity

_____ Reduced platelet count

_____ Slowed inflammatory response

5. Which of the following medications can reduce protein synthesis and cellular growth, thereby reducing the speed of wound healing? Select all that apply.

_____ Antibiotics

_✓_ Steroids

_____ Hypoglycemic agents

_✓_ Chemotherapy agents

_✓_ Antiinflammatory agents

6. Which of the following systemic factors can affect a client's wound healing after surgery?
   a. Body build
   b. Edema
   c. Eschar   } Local factors
   d. Trauma
   e. Sloughing
   f. Infection

7. A client who recently had abdominal surgery has called the nurse to the room to report evisceration. In which position should the nurse put the client?
   a. Prone
   b. Supine
   c. High Fowler's
   d. Low Fowler's
   e. Semi-Fowler's

8. When performing an assessment of a pressure ulcer, the nurse should include what parameters in the assessment?

   Location, size, color, surrounding skin, drainage, temp.)

9. _____ is any soft, pink, fleshy projection that forms during the healing process in a wound that does not heal by primary intention.

10. Indicate whether each of the following statements is true or false.

    a. *False* ___ When caring for a client with a wound bed that presents with a stringy, moist, yellow substance known as slough, it is important to take care not to disturb the tissue.

    b. *True* ___ A moist wound will heal with less scar tissue than a dry, scabbed wound.

11. Match each of the following wound care products with its correct description.

Wound Care Product	Description
a Gauze dressing	a. Water- or glycerin-based; used to maintain wound moisture
d Transparent film	b. Moderately absorptive; can be packed into wounds to promote wound debridement
e Hydrocolloid dressing	
a Hydrogel dressing	c. Forms a soft gel to fill in dead space
c Alginate dressing	d. Allows visualization of the wound
f Foam	e. Promotes autolytic debridement of a necrotic wound
	f. Used on partial- or full-thickness wounds; absorbs drainage around drainage tubes

12. *Debridement* is the removal of dirt, foreign matter, and dead or devitalized tissue from a wound.

13. The physician plans to debride a client's wound. The wound is dressed with a moisture-retentive dressing, creating an occlusive seal. This will allow the macrophages and neutrophils to reduce the necrotic tissue. What type of debridement is being employed in this scenario?
    a. Sharp debridement
    b. Mechanical debridement
    c. Autolytic debridement
    d. Negative pressure debridement
    e. Mechanical debridement

14. The client has developed signs and symptoms consistent with a postoperative wound infection. Which of the following techniques should be used to culture the wound?
    a. Swab the lower aspect of the wound to remove any exudate for a culture.
    b. Swab the center area of the wound to obtain a specimen for a culture.
    c. Swab in a zigzag technique the length of the wound.
    d. Swab the wound at the upper corners to obtain the specimen.

15. Lifestyle factors that can affect a client's surgical prognosis include

    ___nutrition___, ___activity___, ___exercise___, and

    ___substance abuse___.

16. Infants and children have a higher surgical risk than middle-aged adults.
    a. True
    b. False

17. Many herbal remedies may cause adverse effects during and after operative procedures. These must be discontinued during the operative experience to avoid complications. Match each of the following herbal preparations with its physiological effect and the associated complications for surgical procedures.

Herbal Preparation	Preoperative Consideration
_b_ Ginseng	a. Decreases effectiveness of immunosuppressants may cause allergic reactions
_D_ Ginger	b. Has anticoagulant properties; causes hypo-glycemia and edema Antiocoag, ↑BP,↑ Resp.
_C_ St. John's wort	c. May promote possible drug interactions SSRI, MAOI, psychoactive drugs
_A_ Echinacea	d. Associated with prolonged clotting times

18. Which of the following food allergies reported by a client scheduled for surgery may warrant further assessment? (*Hint:* See page 1284 in your textbook.)
    a. Strawberries
    b. Bananas
    c. Iodine
    d. Walnuts
    e. Broccoli
    f. Papaya

19. Match each of the following types of anesthesia with its correct description.

Anesthesia	Description
_c_ Local	a. Produced by inhalation or injection of anesthetic drugs into the bloodstream, causing a loss of all sensation and consciousness
_a_ General	
_e_ Regional	b. Injection of an agent into vessels, producing a lack of sensation over a specific body area
_b_ Nerve block	c. The temporary loss of feeling as a result of the inhibition of nerve endings in a specific part of the body
_d_ Spinal	d. Also known as subarachnoid block; used for surgical procedures on the lower abdomen, perineum, and lower extremities
	e. The instillation of medication into or around the nerves to block the transmission of nerve impulses in a particular area or region

Exercise 2

 CD-ROM Activity

 45 minutes

- Sign in to work at Pacific View Regional Hospital on the Medical-Surgical Floor for Period of Care 1. (*Note:* If you are already in the virtual hospital from a previous exercise, click on **Leave the Floor** and then **Restart the Program** to get to the sign-in window.)
- From the Patient List, select Piya Jordan (Room 403).
- Click on **Get Report** and read the report.
- Click on **Go to Nurses' Station** and then on **403**.
- Click on and review the **Initial Observations** and **Clinical Alerts**.

1. Piya Jordan has an indwelling Foley catheter. Which of the following best explains the rationale for its insertion prior to surgery?
    a. The Foley catheter will allow for close monitoring of urinary output.
    b. Having a Foley catheter will allow the client to rest instead of needing to ambulate to the bathroom or commode.
    c. The Foley catheter will reduce the occurrence of urinary tract infections.
    d. The Foley catheter reduces the size of the bladder and reduces the chance for injury during the surgical procedure.

2. Piya Jordan has a Jackson-Pratt drain. Which of the following statements about this device are correct? Select all that apply.

_____ It was placed in Piya Jordan's incision while she was in the PACU.

_✓_ It will reduce fluid accumulation between surfaces of the wound. *In surgery*

_____ It is a small, pliable, flat latex tube used to promote drainage. — *penRose*

_✓_ It is a closed drainage system.

_____ It is an open drainage system. — *penROse*

_____ It has a cartridge. *Hemovac*

_✓_ It has a bulb.

➤ • Click on **Chart** and then on **403**.
   • Click on and review the **Surgical Reports** and **Physician's Notes**.

3. What surgical procedure was performed on Piya Jordan?

4. Which of the following surgical types describe the procedures performed on Piya Jordan? Select all that apply.

_✓_ Diagnostic

_____ Ablative

_✓_ Palliative

_____ Constructive

_____ Reconstructive

_____ Transplant

5. Piya Jordan had _____ anesthesia.

6. Which of the following terms best describes the urgency of Piya Jordan's surgical procedure?

_____ Elective

_✓_ Urgent

_____ Emergency

7. During the preoperative period, the physician ordered the administration of phytonadione 10 mg SubQ. Why was this medication administered?

→ • Click on and review the **History and Physical** tab.

8. How old is Piya Jordan?

    68

9. Why do older clients have additional risks associated with surgery?

    Impaired circulation, ↓ Renal function,
    ↓hydration/nutrition, thromboemoblic
    complications

10. Piya Jordan's past medical history reflects disorders in which of the following body systems? Select all that apply.

    _____ Pulmonary

    _____ Cardiovascular

    _____ Renal

    _____ Neurologic

    _____ Metabolic

    _____ Integumentary

    _____ Gastrointestinal

    _____ Musculoskeletal

11. Which of the following medications taken by Piya Jordan prior to her hospitalization may be the source of intraoperative and postoperative complications? Select all that apply. (*Hint:* Click on the Drug Guide for assistance.)

    ✓ Digoxin

    ✓ Warfarin

    _____ Celecoxib

→ • Click on and review the **Laboratory Reports** tab.

12. Laboratory testing completed during Piya Jordan's preoperative period reflected some abnormal values. Which of the following laboratory values were abnormal during the preoperative phase? Select all that apply.

    _____ RBC

    _____ INR

    _____ Potassium

    _____ Sodium

    _____ Hemoglobin

    _____ Hematocrit

    _____ Creatinine

    _____ PT

13. What is the most likely reason for Piya Jordan's INR reading?
    a. The history of osteoarthritis
    b. Warfarin therapy at home
    c. History of an irregular heart rate
    d. Constipation

14. For which of the following complications is Piya Jordan at risk because of her INR reading?
    a. Urinary retention
    b. Pneumonia
    c. Paralytic ileus
    d. Hemorrhage

15. Albumin is considered the best indicator of long-term nutritional status. Preoperatively, Piya

    Jordan's serum albumin level was _____ g/dL.

16. Discuss the importance of Piya Jordan's albumin level.

→ • Click on and review the **Physician's Orders** tab.

17. Match each of the following preoperative exercises with the complication(s) they are designed to prevent. (*Note:* Each exercise can have more than one correct answer.)

Exercise	Postoperative Complication
_____ Deep breathing	a. Pneumonia
_____ Coughing	b. Thrombus formation
_____ Turning	c. Atelectasis
_____ Leg exercises	
_____ Incentive spirometry	

18. When should Piya Jordan begin performing postoperative leg exercises?
    a. During the first 24 hours
    b. After the first 24 hours
    c. After the sequential compression devices are discontinued
    d. After the physician institutes ambulation orders

19. Piya Jordan's physician has ordered sequential compression devices. What is the rationale for their use?
    a. To reduce leg cramping
    b. To promote rest
    c. To enhance venous return
    d. To eliminate the occurrence of thrombus formation

→ • Click on **Patient Care** and then on **Physical Assessment** to perform a physical assessment.

20. The assessment of Piya Jordan's chest reveals decreased chest expansion.

    _____Deep_____ breathing will improve her lung expansion and oxygen delivery without using excess energy.

21. When performing the assessment on Piya Jordan's incision, which of the following should be included in the assessment? Select all that apply.

    ___✓___ Approximation of the sutures

    ___✓___ Color of tissue surrounding the incision

    ___✓___ The presence of drainage from the incision

    _____ Total number of sutures

    ___✓___ Odor of the incision

22. During this period in the postoperative phase, Piya Jordan should use a heating pad on her incision to promote comfort.
    a. True
    b. False

23. When caring for Piya Jordan, the nurse should understand that most acute wound infections commonly occur during surgery and within _36_ to _48_ hours after surgery.

24. The manifestations of infection are typically evident within what time period?
    a. 24-36 hours
    b. 24-48 hours
    c. 1-2 days
    d. 2-3 days
    e. 4-5 days
    f. 5-7 days